And So We Heal

Pauline Lomas

It is my simple wish that this book be of Comfort, Hope and Love...

That it serve to give you strength, Almighty power within

First Published 2009 by Appin Press, an imprint of Countyvise Limited.

14 Appin Road, Birkenhead, CH41 9HH

Copyright © 2009 Pauline Lomas

The right of Pauline Lomas to be identified as the author of this work has been asserted by her in accordance with the Copyright, Design and Patents Act 1988.

British Library Cataloguing in Publication Data.
A catalogue record for this book is available from the British Library.

ISBN 978 1 906205 31 7

All rights reserved. No part of this publication may be reproduced, stored in a retrieval system, or transmitted, in any other form, or by any other means, electronic, chemical, mechanic, photograph copying, recording or otherwise, without the prior permission of the publisher.

For my mother, Edna

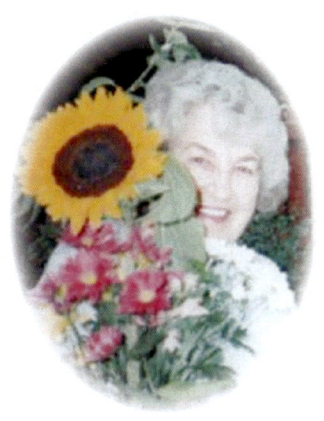

How Blessed I am this day
I have to the best of my ability
produced a book of my journey through healing
to share with others
sisters....brothers
All
To remind us of our indomitable courage. . .
our softness. . .our joy. . .
Indeed, it is our love that shall be reflected back inside
our souls

And we shall heal

~ *And So We Heal* ~

Acknowledgements

Giving birth to a memoir is a curious procedure that begins long before words are put on paper. Mine came welling up from some place deep inside my heart demanding I give it light…How grateful I am then to so very many… A thousand thank yous first and foremost to my mother, my brothers and sisters, my family and my friends for supporting me with their light, their love and their laughter through these long years of healing. I always believed that this book wanted to be written, but writing it at times seemed an overwhelming challenge – more so than, dare I say it, the cancer itself. Without the kindness of my sister Barbara Seddon deciphering and typing up the endless diaries, it would not have been possible to even begin. Another thousand thank yous to my sister artist, Deborah Lomas who was with me on that fateful day of diagnosis, and whose faith in my ability to overcome remained constant, and whose awesome artistic talent continues to inspire me. I am especially grateful to the many friends who gave of their time to read through the various rough drafts and offer wise counsel; Linda Caso, Aurelia Navarro, Steven Carroll, Gerard Rohlfing, Sheila Shaw, Kamila Schertel, Leonie Tremaine, Rosella Longinotti, Jean Gilhead, Adela Bielsa, Gordon Loney, Lou Dunn Diekemper, and Sheila Atkinson, and to Suzanne Lau for her dedication in helping me to put this book together!

A special thank you to Michele Thyne as editor, and to Sue Kernaghan, a survivor herself, working with the NHS as a Macmillan facilitator, for valuable editing, and encouragement.

Thank you to my dear friend Eugene Imai who first brought a healing light from the East into my life, and to the many healing hands whose spirits continue to uplift my own. – And of course 'mil gracias' to Javier who caught the many tears when they fell, and loved them into laughter.

And finally to the ever-present invisible forces at work in all our lives – Bless you all.

~ And So We Heal ~

> "In the heart of the strong shines a
> relentless ray of resolve"

November 2007

"It's remarkable!" The exact words from my Oncologist, Alison Waghorn at the Linda McCartney Clinic in Liverpool, England. What she actually meant was, that it was 'remarkable', because even though I had refused everything offered to me so far; i.e. the conventional-surgery, chemotherapy, radiation, and HRT, my 'cancer marker' and blood tests were showing normal range. It was 'remarkable' because in the six and some years since my breast cancer diagnosis it had not spread to any other part of my body, with the exception of one sentinel node under my right arm, which now seemed to be normal.

REMARKABLE? Yes, I feel pretty remarkable, having lived these past eight years within the mysterious realm of 'cells gone haywire'...

Cancer they called it. I NEVER WOULD!

~ And So We Heal ~

It's almost eight years ago now…unbelievable to me now that it happened - Breast cancer that is. Like a dream…a mystical journey to the depths of my soul…

Although I must tell you this;

I never 'owned' it.

Being told that one has a life-threatening illness such as cancer should be the key for any individual to stop and make some serious life changes. All too often fear can overwhelm and throw us into free-fall where we can become too confused and scared to make our own investigations into the workings of this miraculous body of ours that in truth has just as much power to regenerate as it does to degenerate.

I'm not going to beat about the bush here, but cancer and the process of defeating it is big business. It takes a lot of hard physical and emotional work to tackle disease holistically. Most of us will say we cannot afford to slow down enough to tap into nature's mysterious ways. Modern medicine is wonderful to a point…but many times comes with a price. I did not want to find myself years down the line paying that price, perhaps battling a re-occurrence, which has become widely accepted now as the 'norm'.

So on Thursday October 25th 2001, when I was diagnosed with a malignant 2.5 cm tumour in my right breast, I said no to surgery, radiation and chemotherapy, and decided to follow a natural course of holistic healing. It's not that I wanted to rule out orthodox medicine altogether…indeed no…I wanted to be part of a bridge between the two; walk the middle way, and hopefully find some less invasive way.

~ And So We Heal ~

I wanted to feel good about my choices.

If they came up with something that sounded organically right for me - I'd go for it. It seemed that everywhere I turned folk were dropping by the wayside with these cancer treatments.

Nobody was offering me a sure thing - everything was a risk!

Eradicating this tumour and restoring my immune system to optimum health was my main priority then. It was all about choice and what was intrinsically right for me. Each step upon the journey came from allowing me the time to search within for a truth that had MY name on it.

It is different for all of us, and so I cannot proclaim to hold answers for anyone. I had little money, and so was limited as to what was available to me, but more importantly, I had invested heavily in my spiritual growth over the years, and all the money in the world could not have bought me an ounce of that kind of alchemic gold.

I had enough faith stored up over the years to move a mountain…

So when the still small voice whispered gently in my dreams one night shortly after the horror of being told I had breast cancer, I was aware enough to catch it…

"FIRST DO NO HARM", it said; the wise words of Hippocrates.

~ And So We Heal ~

And so it was I set out in search of healing… natural healing.

I knew without a doubt that my disease had its roots embedded in my own heart-the one that loves forever -The sheer volume of love that had poured forth from this tender vessel over the years was a true testament to what I always believed to be life's purpose…LOVING…

I was proud to count myself amongst the lovers of this world, but what had once kept me alive was now threatening to kill me. Somewhere along the way, all that emotion and passion, all that 'loving to the depths of one's soul', had somehow got tangled up in a ball, and with a series of severe blows upon my psyche had solidified, calcified, inside my breast, bringing my life as it was to a screeching halt. I was no longer available to save anybody's world until I had saved my own.

This was not something the doctors could just cut out and I would return to normal life. I knew instinctively that all was not well in my 'normal' life. The truth is I was sad and heartbroken…Surely there had to be a connection.

It would take time and courage to unravel the toxic mass that had encamped in my breast. Taking time to tune into my own intuition to explore the emotional side of my psyche carved a pathway back through the labyrinth of my life. With careful nutritional guidance and detoxification; confronting life's shadows, delving down deep inside, and beyond ordinary levels of perception, I was able to peel away the layers and connect with a 'higher order of being'…There was nothing else but TRUSTING in the 'all-knowingness' to which there is no name.

~ And So We Heal ~

In the process I began to feel better than I had in years.

Ultimately, the journey has been a rare gift of such spellbinding wonder to me, that I feel destined to share it.

My story does not portend to be a great treatise on the cure for cancer, no great academic achievement to be hailed by science, but hopefully its contents will touch those hearts that chance upon it and help other brave souls on their journey of healing.

Before my diagnosis, I was putting together a book about a very special love story. Guess what? It's still a book about a very special love story...

Beginning then to gather up the thousands of words that lay already written; the diaries…letters…feelings of yesterday, come alive again now. Grasping the golden thread that spins through my life, I attempt to painstakingly weave it into this tapestry, this 'slice of my life', that cries out to be shared.

The Mission then…

To glean…
Re-discover the magic…
Weave the golden thread…
To live...
Simply to live...

And this is my story.

~ And So We Heal ~

Chapter One
Javier & Pauline

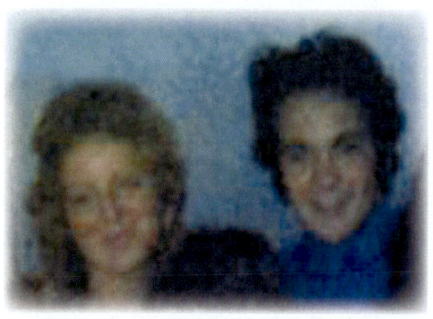

> Life is but a dream,
> And if we are artists then we can create our life with love, and our dream becomes a masterpiece of art.
>
> Toltec

A letter I wrote but never sent…

Dear Javier,

January 3rd 1999
Los Angeles, California

As always, I write from inside my heart, and am grateful to have such a loving friend who can receive my words. Long, long ago I must have been a writer of romance, because my heart thinks always in such ways…and needs to express it.

~ *And So We Heal* ~

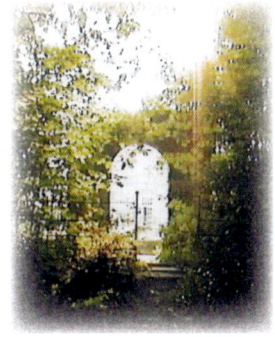

After we spoke today I felt that a door opened through which I can once again send love. I found the story I wrote about us in New York, ONCE UPON A TIME, I called it. We hadn't seen each other for eighteen years then; since Ibiza, remember? I read it and cried. So inspired was I, at seeing you again like that, and realising how much in love I still was with you...but then the terrible knowing that we could not be together...

Writing that story somehow helped me to holdfast...

Even now, whenever I think of you, something beautiful and sweet moves inside me to give me strength. The simple presence of a mystery...

Something that always magically embraces my life when I have needed faith to carry on. I know you have your life with your children, and I could never ask you to give that up...but something inside me is longing to touch you.

How? - I do not know...but I think this longing will just grow and grow until I can.

Perhaps it's an impossible dream...

I am so excited you are painting...Maybe this is your new mission. Flying was just the beginning...

Flying with one's spirit ...now that's something...

Your art... Just imagine all that you can express...giving in to that part of your Self.

That is your magic, your gift! Life begins at fifty...

Wake up and believe that! Don't give in to being old. That is why I came into the world six months after you to keep reminding you. Fight! Fight!

Besos,
Pauline

~ And So We Heal ~

I read somewhere that longing is the deepest and most ancient voice in the human soul. It is the secret source of all presence and the driving force of all creativity and imagination. Longing keeps the door open and calls towards us the gifts and blessings of which our lives dream.

If this is indeed true, I get top marks in longing. Ever since we had met for that first summer on the Spanish island of Ibiza in 1972 I had spent a substantial amount of time over the years doing just that - longing for Javier.

ONCE UPON A TIME was a short story I wrote after seeing Javier again. It had been eighteen years since Ibiza...

Javier Nicolás Infanzón Torre was born in Oviedo, Asturias in Northern Spain in 1951, living the typical country village boy life until his family moved to Barcelona when he was ten years old. I was around ten when my family moved us back to England after years abroad in Malaya as it was then known, and before that Africa. Although our lives touched briefly that summer in Ibiza, our paths were to take very different directions, both marrying other people, and Javier having two children.

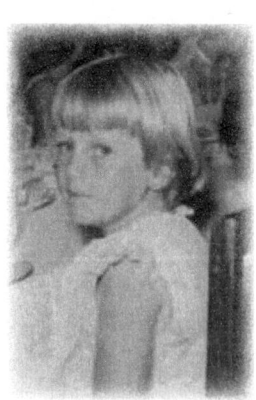
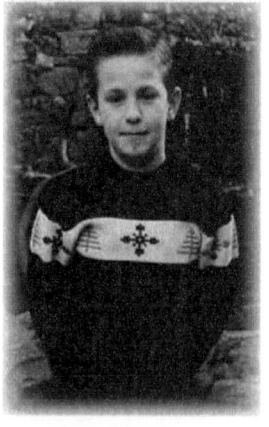

Perhaps it was a romantic yearning for a time of innocence, long since past, that would feed this longing; who can really say. Whatever it was between us certainly had a large role to play in shaping my life...

~ *And So We Heal* ~

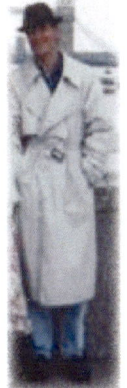

…I mean hello, seeing him again after eighteen years had past, getting out of that cab in New York, with his gabardine and trilby, looking at me like Humphrey Bogart in Casablanca…my long lost love returned!

What was a girl to do? Perhaps I had spent too much time in Hollywood. Destiny may have been conspiring to keep us in touch, but the truth was Javier now had children…he was married!!! There was just no way.

The door closed!

So here I was again in 1999, almost ten years later and not too much had changed in the 'longing' department.

'…Something inside me is longing to touch you.'

Somewhere in that letter lay hidden the key that would unlock the door to our story.
   Something beautiful continued to survive behind that closed door…
   Perhaps it was an impossible dream at that. But the mind is a powerful presence, and love, even more so.
   Long after the portal closed again separating our two worlds, a mysterious web continued to weave us back together…
   Even though I never sent that letter, about fifteen months after I had written those words, fate intervened. Just as my life in America seemed to be dissolving, Javier's too was undergoing major transformation in Spain. Unbeknownst to me at the time his marriage had fallen apart and so had his health. He was living at his mother's house in Barcelona awaiting triple heart by-pass surgery.

~ And So We Heal ~

I had sent him this postcard from the road:

Dear Javier,   *August 15, 2000*
                                           Sedona, Arizona

I am currently flying free…
Gave up my cottage in Sierra Madre and am travelling. I will be in New York- August 23rd- Sept13th with Shumei Taiko, the Japanese drummers, at the United Nations, and various concerts promoting Peace. Then on to my mother's home in the UK - Probably through October, and then-? I hope you are strong and bright and your family is well.
I am fine now - but I've had a very strong purification for my soul.
I am much better now.
Keep painting…
Love, Pauline

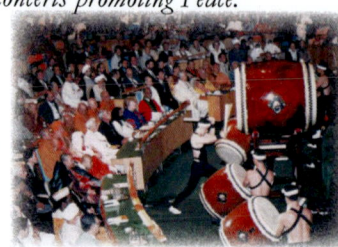

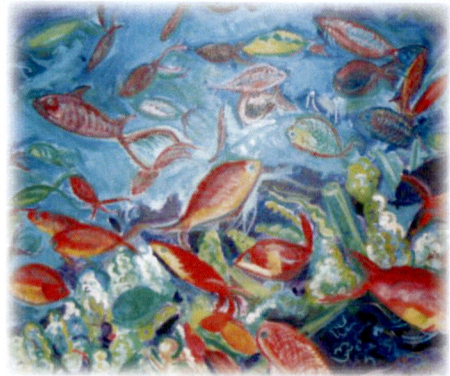

'Keep painting…'

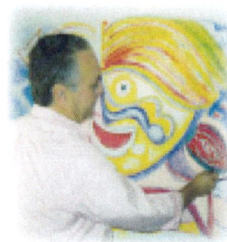

It seems that we both had changed course and started painting at the same time. That's what I had been doing since giving up my career as an actress following the death of my partner Tom, in 1996. My first book

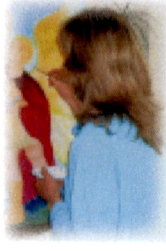

~ *And So We Heal* ~

'*Bridges, a Memoir of Love*', based on the diary I kept whilst working on the film '*The Bridges of Madison County*', chronicles our story – more about that later.

It was a time of major transition. Being cast as the voice of Alicia Masters in the 'Fantastic Four' animation series on television was a final lucky break for me but when that concluded and Tom lost his battle with cancer, I didn't have the heart for Hollywood anymore and had retreated into the woods of Sierra Madre - California, painting and becoming increasingly involved in projects that nurtured a more peaceful existence…It's such a cliché, but the way I saw things; all roads needed to lead to love…

'Love is always the message!' End of story!

In 1996 as both a form of grief therapy, and needing to earn a living, I began creating a line of glass art specifically designed to inspire, and heal, beginning with the first ´Chalice of Light', with the word 'Believe' inscribed on it. Surprisingly, or not…there in my cabin…my 'Lovelands', as it was aptly called, I became enamoured with working in this way… My creativity was fulfilled and my broken heart healed…. or so I thought.

When a canyon fire threatened to destroy my cottage in Sierra Madre, and seven deer were found impaled on an iron rod fence, having attempted to leap over it, I could sense that a foreclosure to my 'life as it was'; was imminent, and though I clung to it for dear life, reflecting back it feels as if some mighty force came and ripped me out of there.

For a while, I was lost in the woods. Finding my way back, I believe I was very much helped by 'Jyorei', a healing light technique meaning 'purification of the spirit' which I had practiced for years. Similar to Reiki and having its roots in Japan; Jyorei and the fellowship of Shumei had become an important part of my life. I've told the story so many times that I fear it may have lost some of it's lustre. But the truth is in 1983 after many years of trying to succeed with my acting career I found myself on my knees one-day praying to God to get me out of Hollywood. Imagine my surprise then when I heard a knock on the door and opened it to find a very sincere looking Japanese man.

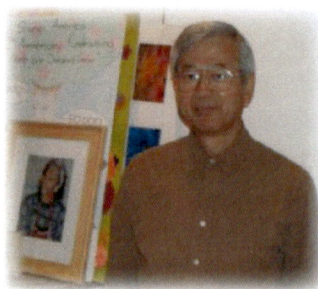

"Hello my name is Eugene Imai and I am here to pray for your health and happiness?" he said; so very polite and sincere in his manner. I agreed to receive **this Jyorei, this special ray of light channelled for my well-being.** How on earth could I possibly refuse when I had without doubt been imploring the grace of God just moments before?

There is more to healing than repairing broken bones.
Healing is about mending broken hearts and calming agitated minds. Most importantly it is about renewing the spirit…'
Jyorei… "An offering of Light"
by Roy Gibbon and Atsushi Fujimaki

My life was about to be transformed and within a year my wish was granted when I found myself on top of a mountain in Japan with a hundred taiko

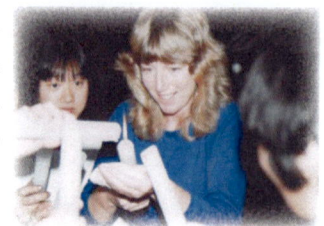

16

drums being beaten in celebration as a rainbow appeared mystically around the sun; but that is another story.

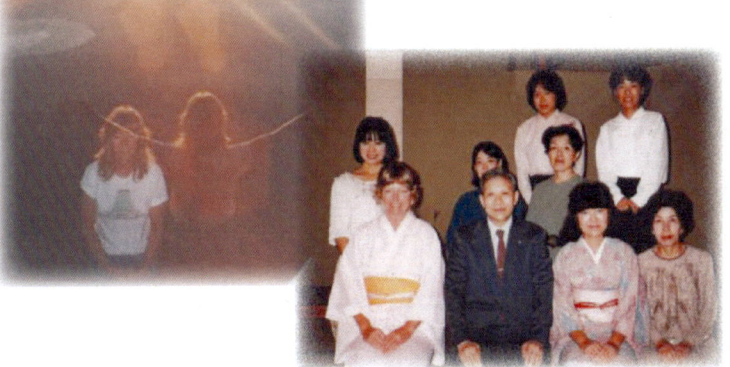

Here I was all these years later undergoing more 'purification'. The year before I had travelled to South Africa with the drummers narrating for them at the 'Parliament of the Worlds Religions'. This mystical drumbeat is world-renowned and can affect profound healing. Drumming has been a necessary and respected skill amongst holy women throughout history. In my case, I really feel that it helped to drum me back in some way.

I wrote this about Africa:

When Koji Nakamura, leader of the Shumei Taiko Ensemble, asked me to introduce and narrate their performances at the Parliament of the World's Religions in Cape Town, South Africa, I immediately agreed... Driving from the airport past the shanty towns, where the poorest of the poor have created a community from which to dream of a better life, I began to release my own fears of lack - and suddenly the $50 dollars I had in my pocket seemed like a million.

...After a few hours' sleep I awoke to witness a brilliant red sun from my hotel window and a giant statue of an Angel reaching up from

~ And So We Heal ~

down below. Mr. Nakamura came to my room for what was to be an everyday ritual of chanting and exchanging Jyorei. The energy was very strong within him and I witnessed a strong flash of purple light around his head. I was in the presence of a master spirit.

…Whilst the drummers continued with their rigorous training and long distance running I, too, would rise early and take brisk walks through the city, allowing the words that preceded each drum piece to find an organic pacing. Talking in front of hundreds and sometimes thousands of people meant that I, too, must focus. As with my painting, I needed to be both spontaneous and yet plugged into a cosmic consciousness. It could not be simply a performance- it needed ritual, and that only came through with permission from a higher source, that I knew. I learned so much from the discipline of the drummers and would awake in the early hours, my eyes filled with tears of joy and understanding. I knew that it was a combination of many, many candles gathered together to produce one light that was affecting me so, but I could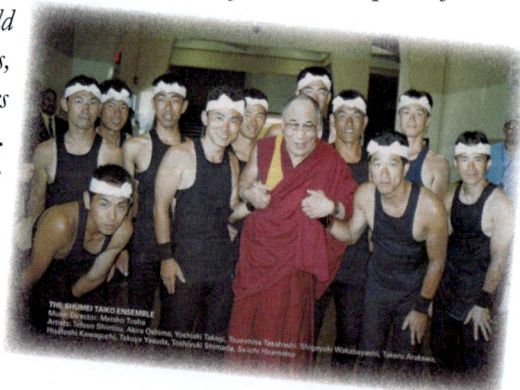
not deny the way the drumbeat was quickening me, altering my breath so that I could breathe deeply and easily, and with that deeper remembering of who I am at soul level.

18

~ And So We Heal ~

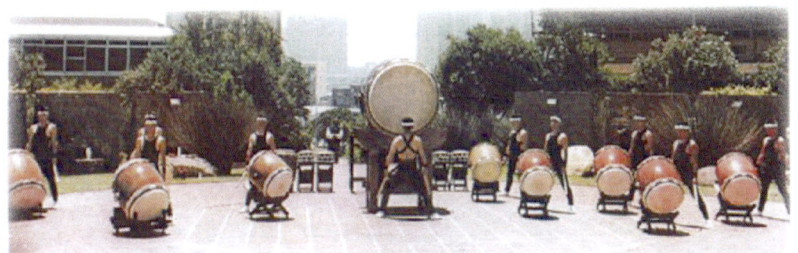

photographs by Rose

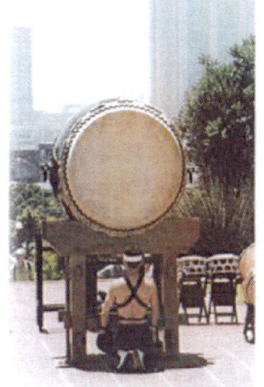

The mystical power
which springs
from the artist's soul
passes through
the written word
through the visual image
the musical instrument
the song or dance
and plucks at the soul
of all mankind.

~ Mokichi Okada

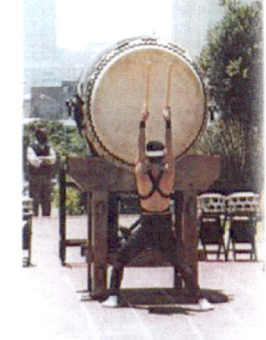

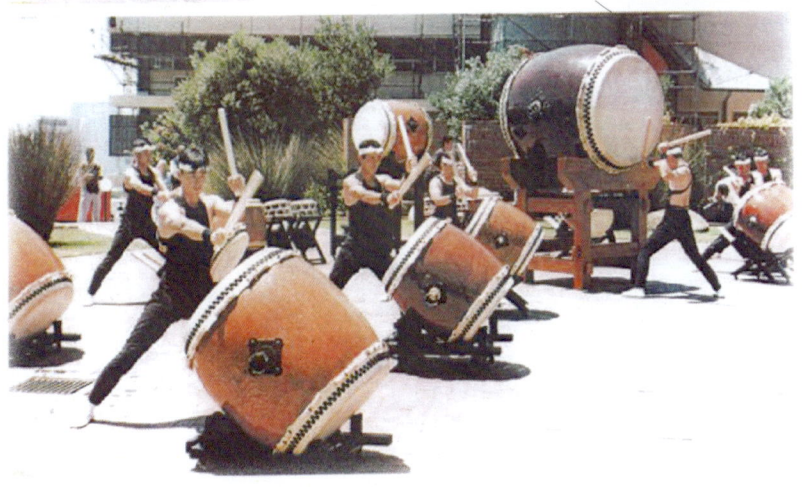

~ *And So We Heal* ~

So when Javier called to tell me of his forthcoming 'heart-by-pass' operation it was October 2000 and I had literally just arrived in England from America, where I had been with the drummers again at the United Nations for The Millennium Peace gathering. I remember feeling very much empowered with a sense of some new beginning but not really sure of what life held in store for me. Since dissolving my household in California I had reluctantly bought a mobile phone so as to at least keep in touch with friends and not get too lost in the woods; but the battery having barely lasted the transatlantic crossing was just about to die when I discovered Javier's voice in the message box. He had been trying to find me - our postcards it seems had crossed in the mail.

Our lives were shifting once more and we were reaching out to each other again…

Dear Pauline, *September 30th,*
2000 Barcelona
…I've been trying to find you…the doctors are going to make some by-pass in my heart this October, but I'm all right…hoping for a quick recovery-
…Send the next letter to my mother's house. I'll be there.
Besos, Javier

Some by-pass in his heart!!!

My God! Javier certainly had a way with words. Although I didn't know it at the time, he had actually been declared dead at one point.

It's over forty years now...our friendship...our being 'amantes', 'star-crossed lovers'. There has always been a 'Darling Javier' snuggled inside my mind; destiny, somehow managing to keep us apart, but now, ironically, our lives were mirroring each other's. We were both returning 'home to the womb' in a way.

The portal had indeed opened again...

Within a week I found myself in Javier's arms, in Barcelona.

'When are you coming to Barcelona?' he asks.
'Every day, every day', I say.
'I come to Barcelona every day in my mind.'
June 15, 1992, California

Barcelona
I have always had a deep affinity for Spain. Amongst my earliest memories as a child, when we lived in Wales, is visiting our Spanish neighbours whose way of life held me spellbound. Later upon returning home I would entertain myself by dancing through the house singing at the top of my voice in Spanish. The Doris Day hit – 'Que Sera Sera' – 'Whatever will be, will be...the future's not ours to see...' or....Canta no llora... 'Sing, don't cry' were amongst the many favourites that drove my parents crazy.

Of all the cities in my life, it is Barcelona that has revealed to me the 'Portal' of which I have so often spoken. My roots are in England where I was born. I've lived in Africa, Malaysia, America and Japan, but it is here behind the wooden shutters sheltered from a hot Spanish sun that so much of my heart would come to be healed...

~ And So We Heal ~

Now, all these years later in 2000 when Javier came to meet me at the airport there was no denying that we were no longer the fresh-faced teenagers of our long ago youth. But all the same when we fell into each others arms it was as if we were breaking through a spell, and there inside some secret hiding place in our never-ending story, not a moment had been lost.

The diaries I kept help me now to gather fragments... layers...gossamer veils of finely woven memories...

October 9, 2000, Columbus Day, Barcelona.
Once more I am blessed with miracles in my life... By none other than Divine Grace I am here with Javier, a twin-soul, without doubt. How the mysteries have drawn us together over the years is something sacred to me and always shall be.
He is scheduled to undergo triple heart-by-pass surgery in the next two weeks. Seeing him again awakens sweetness in my own heart...
We began our story over thirty years ago... both eighteen, living on the
  Spanish island of Ibiza. I remember looking down from my window one day and seeing this beautiful young man...my heart stirred. We were young and carefree then, and our destinies would lead us far apart...It is only now, in reflecting upon our friendship, that I can recognise him as my 'Anam Cara', a Gaelic word meaning 'friend of the soul' - someone to whom you can confess the hidden intimacies of your life - to whom you can share your innermost self, your mind and your heart.

You are joined in an ancient way to this friend of your soul.

With my days here in Barcelona I seek to remember far beyond ordinary perception. I seek to discover yet another golden key that shall help me to repair the wounds of my friend, my 'Anam Cara', my

Javier...and with that, also heal any unforgiven chasms of pain and guilt that lie dormant within the story of 'us'.

Making love with Javier carries me as always to deep mysterious places...

His kisses soften the screams and torment of recent months when I sought to rip myself free from the America that has been home for the past twenty-five years.

Our seeking to explore those dark forgotten places of body and soul give birth to the release of a throbbing ecstasy that has slowly been emerging as a ball of light inside my soul.

In truth, I have been yearning for Javier...not knowing how or when I would ever see him again... Now as if in my dreams I am here in the arms of the 'Beloved'; that which has never ceased to love me through the absence, the pain, the distance of years...I am here simply to pray for his heart, for his new 'self'...

Not knowing why we are together like this, and not knowing for how long...it is enough then to just live in the moment – magically - en carpe diem.

What did I tell you about the longing!

There was much to heal between Javier and me. He had kept all my letters and postcards to him over thirty years. In reading them I began to understand the depth of my love for him, and re-connect with a part of myself that I had lost.

There is this alchemy between us that seems to awaken something primordial. As teenagers, it was the awakening of this 'life-force' that drew us together, although I remember always trying to suppress my sexual yearnings then. Javier represented the promise of some forbidden treasure that I must resist. In that way, I suppose our relationship was very innocent, never going beyond kissing and cuddling.

~ And So We Heal ~

Over the years, we would go on to lead very different lives. Mine would transport me far away to America, to Hollywood to pursue a life-long dream. He stayed in Europe, worked for his father and became a helicopter pilot; married and had two children.

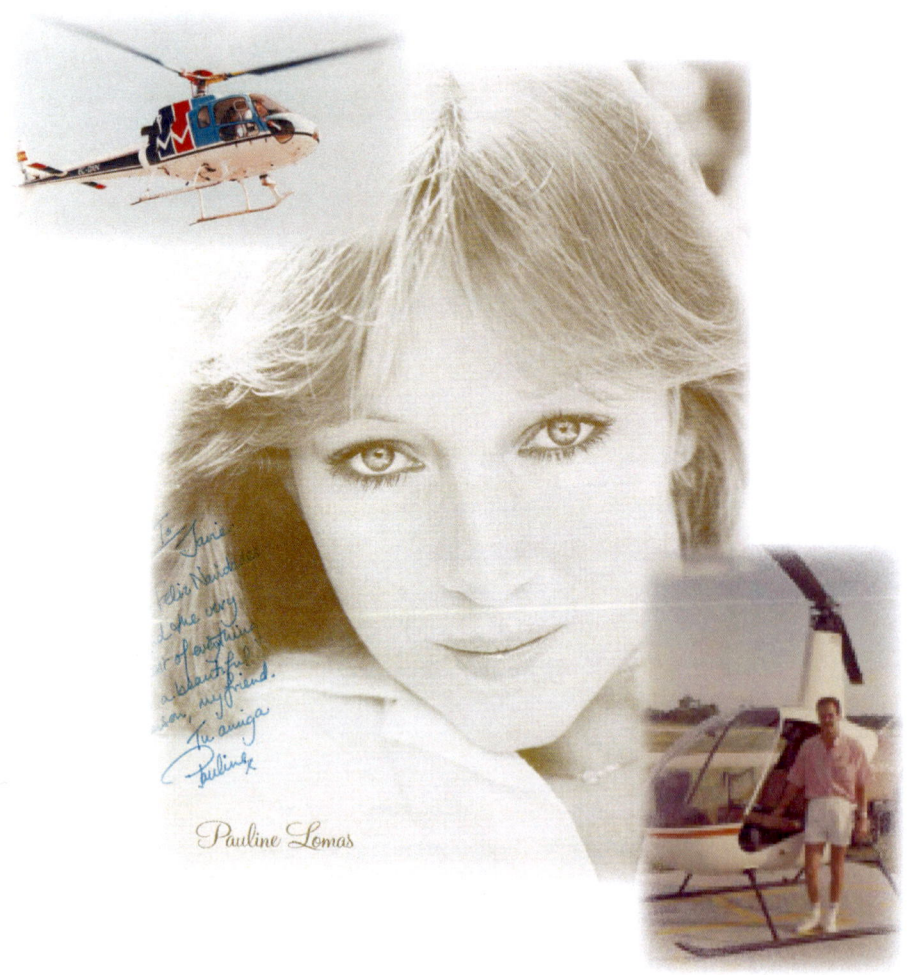

Pauline Lomas

~ *And So We Heal* ~

In 1976 he contacted me again and I wrote this back:
Dear Javier,
...So much seems to have happened in my life especially this last year. I've been living in the U.S.A for the past three years. I was married to a guy from Uruguay until we moved to California and I started drama school (my life-long dream) In the process I was getting in touch with myself and learning to love life and make the most of everything especially my career. I guess my husband couldn't quite understand the change I was going through and we grew further and further apart, until we eventually separated. It was painful at first but I grew to enjoy my independence once again and felt like a bird being set free from her cage. I'm studying at the Lee Strasberg Theatre Institute and love every minute of it. I have beautiful friends and am extremely happy and positive. Being an actress is the number one thing in my life, and living in California is so wonderful. One of these days you'll see me smiling down at you from a stage or screen. It could be next year, or it could be ten years from now, it really doesn't matter – I have direction at last...

A bird being set free...
Obviously I was enjoying this new direction in my life after years of being in an oppressive marriage. It was true...I was completely dedicated to my career as an actress, and was studying at one of the best theatrical schools of its day. I was so determined in those early days. I was twenty-four years old and about to take Hollywood by storm..........Or so I thought!

At the end of my letter I write: '*...you are always welcome at my door.*' and I meant it. But the truth was that it would take many more years before that day would arrive.

Javier's life was moving in another direction. At the age of twenty-four he was about to become a father.

~ *And So We Heal* ~

And so it was… we were living such different lives over the many years… occasionally weaving back together to touch that something special - to know that it still existed. To know that whatever it was that had first blossomed between us had a mysterious never-ending life of its own.

God knows I had done my best to lay this longing to rest, yet somehow, somewhere in the embers of this forbidden love grew a 'yearning' that I could once again connect with.

It was all quite evident now re-reading some of these many letters I had written over the years. I make no apologies any more for the words that came forth then …I was once a romantic storyteller remember?

And I was living my dream in Hollywood.

May 5, 1992, Hollywood, California

Dear Javier,

It is 5.35am, and the falling rain on my balcony has awakened me. The birds are singing very happily and loudly. It is dawn and the streetlights are still on, as I sit in my bedroom writing to a beautiful man whom I cannot forget…I see his face everywhere.

Since I watched you pass through the airport doors that would take you back to your world, I try hard to return to mine; but I keep looking for your arms, your lips, your breathing, next to mine…I keep listening for your words, and the feeling of love that I know shall never fade. Your kisses are the same as they were when first we ever kissed, and now as I write this letter, the tears are falling from my eyes…

I wanted to write something funny, but I must put these memories on paper now whilst I am somewhere between our worlds. All too soon I must pass through the portal to my other world…

My flight back to America was fine…I relived all the moments we shared, and I thought of all the things I did not say. I know I said

~ And So We Heal ~

the most important ones and I hope you realise how much I mean it.

Seeing you again this time has left such a profound feeling in my heart and soul...I cannot really understand it, but this I know...

I love you more than I have ever loved any man, and if it were not for your circumstances, I would move Heaven and Earth just to be with you.

If I could make a wish come true it would be to wake up to your smiling face every day...to take care of you...to grow old with you... in a garden.

Maybe one-day...Que sera, sera...

I wanted you to know these things because of all the past times in 'our story', when I wanted you, and you wanted me, but we never had the right timing.

Please take care of yourself, especially your health...I cannot begin to think of my life without you in it, no matter how far apart life may keep us. There has been too much pain in my life. If I lost you, I would lose my will to continue on. It's as if you and I are a kind of mirror...

Anyway...I am writing too much of sad things...I must start to be happy now and remember our laughter...we always have lots of that.

So...I must get out of this bed now, and begin to find my life in Hollywood again.

You are forever in my heart, and I am always here if you need me.

Pauline

It was true…all true…

Shortly after this Javier wrote to tell me his father had died.

~ And So We Heal ~

Just over two months later I am writing this:

July 23, 1992, UK
Dear Javier,
My father died on Monday July 20th, and I am in England with my family. It is very sad and at one moment I am crying, and the next I am at peace. He was a good man, and of course I am wishing I could have been with him more: but he is finally free from the pain of his physical body. I know his spirit is with us...I can feel his strength. This life is so short....
I hope you are well and happy. I will stay here until September, and when everything is calmer I hope to fly to Majorca or somewhere. I hope to see you.

Your friend, Pauline

Our lives were mirroring each other's again. We did see each other that same summer. I flew to Piedra Llaves, a small village close to Avila in Spain, where Javier was flying helicopters. It was such an emotional journey for us both at that time, having just lost our fathers, and finding ourselves back in each other's arms.

August 17, 1992, Piedra Llaves, Spain
...I've climbed high on to a mountaintop, trying to escape my thoughts, but they follow me everywhere. Below the sounds of the toreadors echo from the bullring. We are at the end of a three-day fiesta and the bulls are being fought and slaughtered. It is the custom in Spain and I try to accept it. There is so much in life I try to accept...bringing me to the question of Javier. Over the last four years he has become increasingly important in my life again, in ways I do not fully comprehend. I see

~ And So We Heal ~

his eyes everywhere. *When I smile, it is his smile; when I shed tears they are for him… When I am with him I long to be with him always.*

What a wonderful gift I have been given…to come back in time and love like this, sharing the magic of our hearts – this love that refuses to die – this friendship that keeps beckoning from far far away.

…The other day he told me that part of his spirit feels as if it has died, that there is emptiness, a lack of direction about what lies ahead in his life.

I feel the same. Of course we are both in mourning for our fathers, and there is so much going on in his personal life with the children, and I try to understand what it is like to be him.

I do not desire to take him away from them, but whether I like it or not **I somehow know that I am forever part of his life, as he is part of mine…**

These few days together were more significant than I could know yet.

Here in these mystical mountains around Avila, amidst prayers for the dead, and ecstasy for the living I remember one day finding myself in a small village church lighting candles to the image of a beautiful Madonna that held me transfixed. I was secretly yearning for a child, so in love was I with Javier.

My prayers were answered…

When I returned to America I found that I was pregnant.

Because of the fact that Javier was already married with two children and the whole idea of possibly tearing a family apart; a decision was made to terminate the pregnancy. It was not something I undertook lightly and for years I have revisited the whys and wherefores of such a decision.

Let us suffice to say that an iron door slammed that day - a wound was registered although I could not see it. There would be others. That is life. I find no words in my diary to help me describe what I was feeling until this several months later:

October 1, 1992, California
The pain and sorrow subside.
They must, so that I can go on living.
I must live this new life with courage.
A beautiful white angel appeared in the sky today-
I know that God is with me…

Javier and I would not see each other again for eight years… There would be many more tears yet to cry… I took these words of the thirteenth century poet Rumi to heart:

> One day your heart will take you to your lover.
> One day your soul will carry you to your beloved.
> Don't get lost in your pain.
> Know that one-day your pain will become your cure.

Little did I know.

~ And So We Heal ~

Chapter Two
Tom's Story

> Tears are a river that takes you somewhere. Weeping creates a river around the boat that carries your soul-life. Tears lift your boat off the rocks, off dry ground, carrying it down river to some place new, some place better.
>
> Clarissa Pinkola Estés

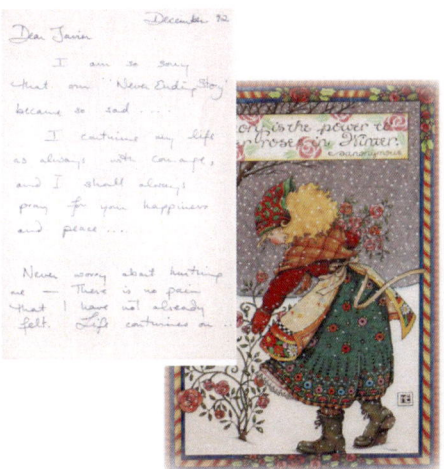

I wanted to be with Javier so much at that time, but I had to somehow put his memory to rest. He was not free; he had a life in Spain; there were children, and so my conscience would not allow me to dream freely of his love. The short-lived reunion in Spain was a gift from God. If I am honest, I put others needs before my own and did what I thought was morally correct.

The door was closed again, or so I thought.

My life had to move forward - there would be journeys yet to make for me and loves to love.

~ And So We Heal ~

Tom came into my life firstly to make me laugh. We were two very sad souls when we met; each confiding our deepest hurts. It was with some reluctance on my part that we became lovers, as Tom was in a marriage, albeit an unhappy one. I had asked for some kind of guidance from God that our relationship was meant to continue. The answer came in a dream in which I saw very clearly a golden angelic form floating above me. 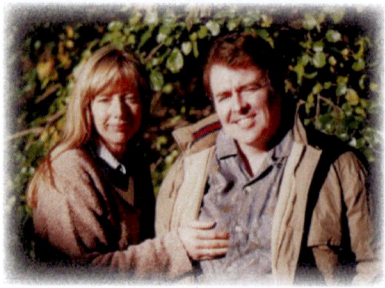 It hovered there for some time then descended into me, and whispered that I should indeed give Tom the love he needed. Shortly after that Tom was diagnosed with cancer. I documented his journey on video and in a little book I wrote in 1995. - Bridges a Memoir of Love. Tom died in 1996.

...Years later, in 2002, I would write this in my diary:

My sister, Deborah and I went to see the new film about Virginia Woolf, 'THE HOURS'. It was quite extraordinary really especially watching Meryl Streep. Her image brought back so many memories and desires to create a piece of work that can touch others as this has touched me.

Ironically, later that evening I watched 'THE BRIDGES OF MADISON COUNTY', on television. It was on very late and part of me fought hard NOT to watch it, fearing that I would be drawn back to re-visit the past I suppose, but somehow getting drawn in all the same. Each frame held a specific meaning for me since I helped to create it in a way. It would be the last film I ever worked on.

~ And So We Heal ~

How strange to watch it and see Meryl on the screen but feel my own body and invisible image there too…like an imprint, a ghost…a haunting…

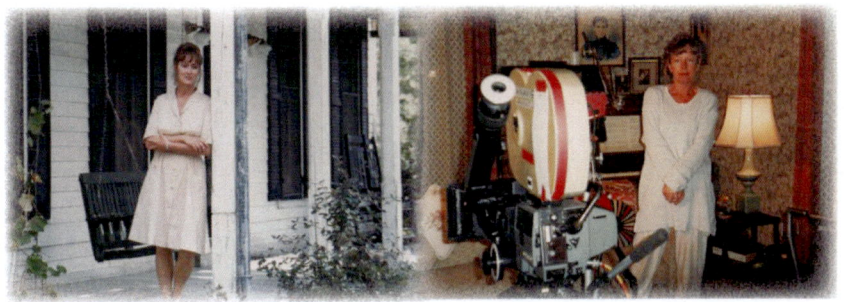

It was the music that struck the deepest. Those few simple keys magically played on the piano unlocked a part of my heart that I had buried. Tears sprang from my eyes and I allowed myself to travel back along those dusty roads to Madison County, to Francesca's house, to the people of Iowa, to Clint tinkling this very tune on the piano as I happened to pass by one lunch hour. To all those memories we built around a story that, in fact was not real.

Choices…it was all about these choices that were made between two lovers and how their lives would forever be affected.

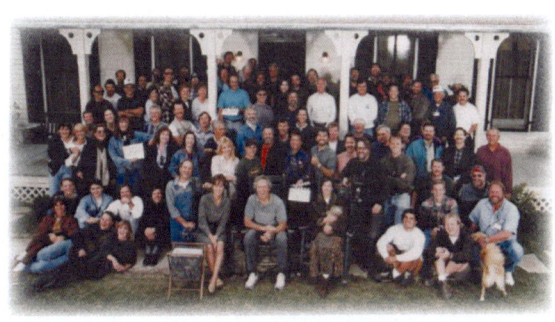

The reality however was that Francesca and Robert did not exist except within the pages of a tiny book, and consequentially on film; but so many lives were touched because of their story.

A year or so after the film opened I found myself back there with Tom. He was born in Iowa. I had written my own book revolving

~ And So We Heal ~

around my work on the film, and the journey through Tom's cancer, BRIDGES, A MEMOIR OF LOVE.

Publishing the book was my giving birth to a dream of sorts I suppose...the child I never had. Returning to Iowa, signing books at 'Roseman Bridge', being there with Tom was completing a circle in a way.

Francesca and Robert could not be together...Tom and Pauline still were...But in truth they were marching towards his death.

I returned to Los Angeles leaving Tom in Iowa so that he could visit his relatives. A few days later when I picked him up at the airport, there was a strange black cloud hanging over our every move. The engine of my car literally caught fire and died as I pulled in to the airport parking lot; and the next day Tom was in so much pain with his breast that he went to the doctor, and begged the surgeon to cut it off.

It's all so symbolic to me now when I look back, as I fight so hard to keep my own breast...

Tom was a 'beloved' on the path...You know the song... 'If you can't be with the one you love, love the one you're with', that was Tom. He literally walked on to a stage in front of me as I sat for the first time in Sheree North's acting class; late as I remember; and making everyone laugh...that was Tom.

How I wanted him to stay here on the earth so that we could live the 'happily ever after' story that I felt was owing to us.

Looking back, I see us as part of a dream that was never going to materialise, as we would wish... But we had a damn good time of it all... capturing so much of our life on video; ever determined to

34

break down the walls of Hollywood. But since we ran out of time on the Hollywood dream, it was our own life story that would be the big 'drama' we would star in. There was lots of love, and that's more than a lot of people get.

THE BRIDGES OF MADISON COUNTY was the last film I ever worked on.

When Tom died, most of my dreams died too.

I realised years ago that my dream to become a famous actress was simply some youthful yearning that had attached itself to my psyche, as a burning ambition to prove myself to the world. Through the art of acting, I learned to exercise 'imagination', and through my exploration of the 'magical' I began to find the essence of who I really am.

There is a deep need inside of me to create something to inspire others…to touch them, to help them open their hearts…ultimately…to the Divine… to that place in the heavens that resonates with the human heart.

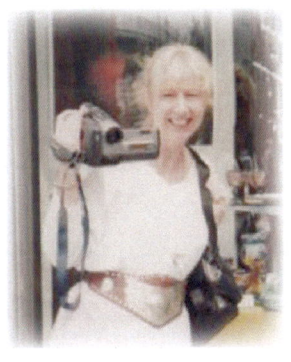
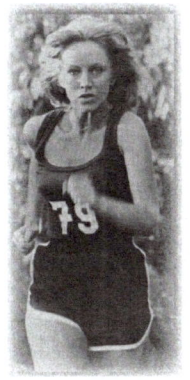
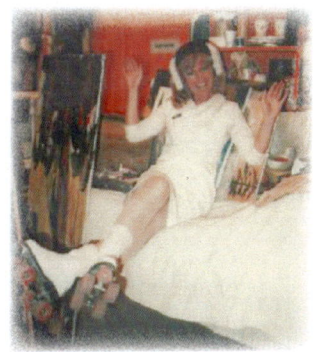

~ And So We Heal ~

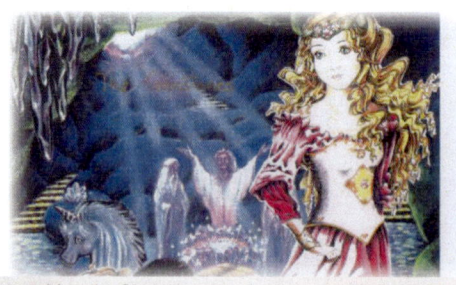

In searching to find the star inside myself I naturally gravitated towards Hollywood and re-discovered that delicate instrument keeping us all alive..The Heart. I've never had any problem giving mine, but the pain of picking up the pieces after it was torn apart several times forced me to look a little deeper into this thing called love.

Thus my dream was born right here in a town so very often labelled 'loveless'; and the beginning of my love-hate relationship with Hollywood. I am by nature a survivor, but only through intense love and belief that our dreams can come true could I have come this far; and only with more of the same can I expect to go further........... and I will

..........with all my heart,

Lets dream upon forever
For ever dreams come true
They may not last forever
For that is up to you.

THE GEMSTONES
TM
Copyright Oct. 16, 1989

Opening... Instrumental

Vocal..."Dream with us" (2 or 3 lines)
Dream with us beyond the world of never
Where magic kingdoms full of light give peace

Narrator... Once upon the eternity of time there was peace and happiness, and joy filled the hearts of all humankind. Deep below the earths surface, 'The Gemstones', slept peacefully, dreaming of a world in harmony.

... Music underscore begins to change from light to dark...

Narrator... With the passing of time came change....and dark forces of illusion began to stir. What once was peaceful became troubled (thunder). What once was happy became sad (effects). The true meaning of love was lost somehow like a distant memory. Cries for help to save mother earth echoed through-out the world awakening 'The Gemstone family.' The time had come for them to help restore the peace that once was.

~ And So We Heal ~

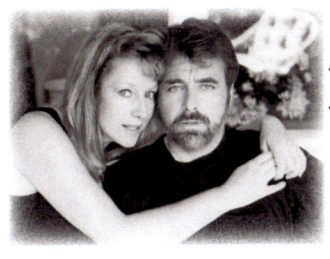

After losing Tom I was mysteriously guided to begin painting glass, as a form of grief therapy. As an artist, albeit a grieving one, I somehow had license to inhabit the invisible realms, and for many years the *'CHALICES OF LIGHT'*, and later the *'TOUCHSTONES'*, I created, became the vessels of my Love and faith in the good things of this world.

I've put my paintbrush away for the most part and picked up my pen again. Since I must continue to nurture a livelihood in order to survive I have no choice but to heed that 'still small voice' once more.

"Take them back to the bridge", I hear Tom say, and see his image talking to Wyman, the good man that owns the gift shop there. Thousands still make the pilgrimage to the bridge to pay homage to a simple 'love story'.

Perhaps he's right; perhaps that's where I must go with this…full circle.

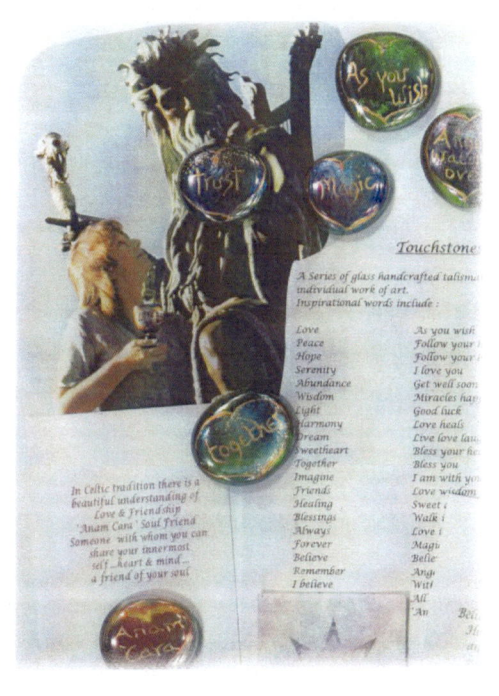

Tom and I came together to heal our wounded hearts. 'Love' came as a beautiful gift even as it was carried on the wings of death.

But Tom was just one chapter in my life.

It would be one year after Tom died that I would hear from Javier again; his heart had stopped and he had almost died.

~ And So We Heal ~

Javier had been the wound that Tom came to heal.
Now it was Javier returning to heal the wound of losing Tom.
Slowly…very slowly, our hearts began to beat together again… through distance and time…

The portal was opening…

It seems there has always been a whisper that says "Javier".

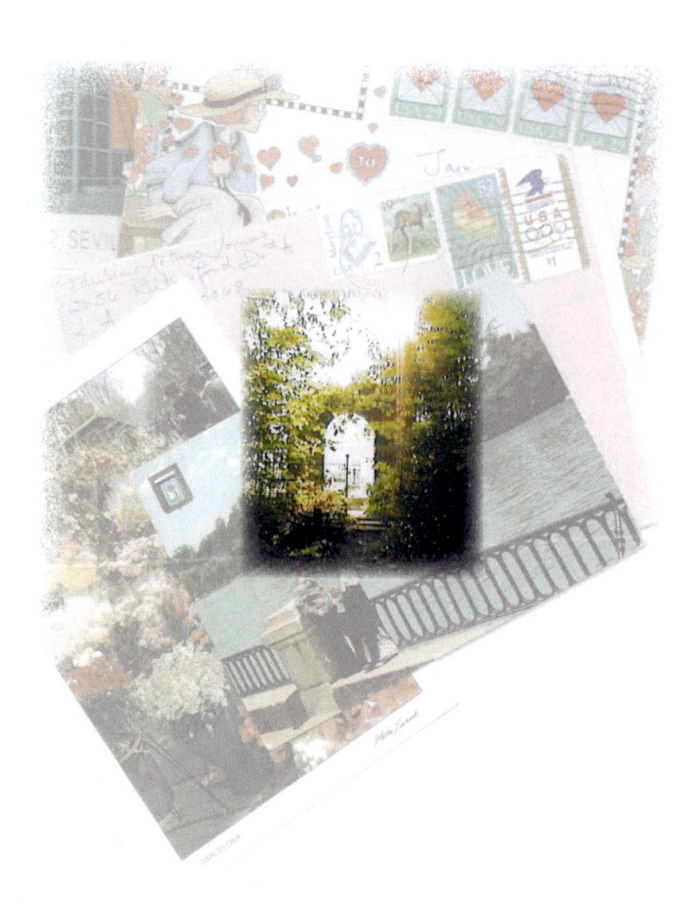

Chapter Three

¡Que Sera Sera!

> Redemption heals a once open wound. But there will be a scar, nevertheless. With changes of weather the scar can and will ache again. That is the nature of a true grief.
>
> Clarissa Pinkola Estés

So finally after all that longing someone must have been listening because here I was in Barcelona with Javier. Once again it was the dreamer that held my pen hostage using words like 'golden keys', and 'Divine Grace', encouraging my spirit to dream again of what could be.

Que sera sera!...whatever will be will be...

…The future was not ours to see. The truth was, Javier was seriously ill awaiting the by-pass that could give him a new lease on life, albeit one depending on a lifetime of medicine. It was such a bittersweet time.

October 12, 2000, Barcelona
Life seems so very fragile at the moment…
Everything hanging in the balance.
It's my first day without Javier by my side so

~ And So We Heal ~

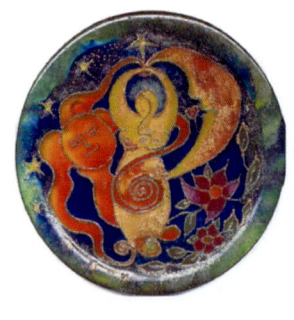

I feel a little lost and sad at first but slowly through writing and painting I re-connect with my essence, having mined the gold for which my heart has been yearning.

Later I enjoy sitting outside a café in the local neighbourhood close to Parc Guell, Gaudi's masterpiece. Sipping on a 'café con leche', writing in my diary; all fit my spirit so well...

There's a need to be close to Javier's physical body at this time, afraid that I might lose him again. I even went to the Cathedral and lit a candle. The statue of Jesus with sacred heart shining so brightly, would ordinarily seem quite garish, but somehow now it gave me peace of mind.

October 15, 2000, Barcelona

I'm sitting in the Plaza Del Pi in old town. The sun is out after two days of rain. Yesterday I painted all day and am happy with the chalices and other pieces I am creating.

The ambience here in Barcelona warms me so very much and being close to Javier is becoming even sweeter. Last night he brought me some of the letters that I have written to him over the many years. I stayed up all night reading them and realized that this love I have for him has been with me all along, despite the many sacrifices I felt that I had to make because of our circumstances.

Life here in Europe is so radically different to that in America. I've got my appetite back and am enjoying the Mediterranean food. There's a wedding taking place here in the Plaza, with musicians playing and people strolling through the network of tiny alleyways in old town.

I find myself wanting to return here to paint and write. When I first arrived back in England after America I had no idea what direction

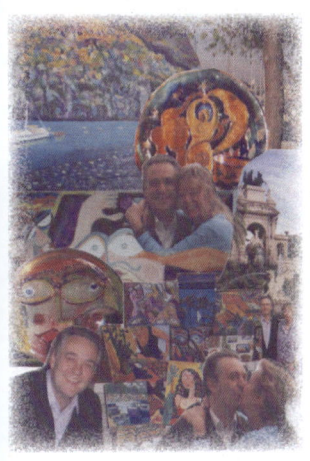

my life was going to take; but now something stirs in my heart again…
I recognize it as hope.

The portal seems to have opened allowing Javier and I this time together. Rather than fear for his operation I *must* believe that all shall be well. There is a difference in him since I came; the colour in his face, his smile.

New blood is pumping through his heart and through mine for that matter.

…Whispers of hidden things that I hesitate to speak of… they float like baby feathers falling from the heavens… Celestial secrets from the gods.

October 17, 2000, Barcelona

It's my ninth day here and I *must now prepare to go to London for a few days then back to my mother's house. I wish I could stay indefinitely* but we know now that the operation is at least two or three weeks away, maybe more and I need to be making money. It's as simple as that.

This afternoon as I sat painting, my eyes met with a huge white feather floating down from the heavens outside my window. I paused breathing in the silent significance- I had just painted the word 'Hope' on a chalice… my mind was playing with words…'La Copa d'esperanza.' 'The Chalice of Hope'

Disappointed at not actually being able to catch the feather, I had continued painting when from the corner of my eye I saw the tiniest of feathers appear … from out of thin air it came…floating directly into the palm of my hand, which held the cup.

~ And So We Heal ~

How can I possibly explain to anyone
These things that appear in my life
To give me the strength to believe?
How can I repay these miracles of nature?
That my soul be so touched
And my head turn about the room
Searching…
For the invisible angels I know
stand guard upon my life.

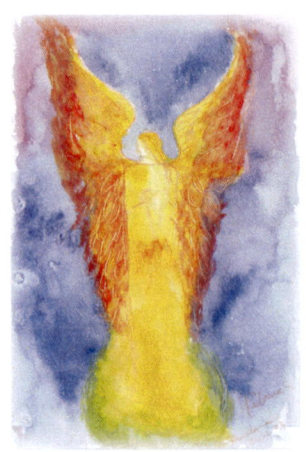

Now three hours later, I have taken a walk and am eating a 'bocadillo con queso' and café con leche. I open this book to write down my thoughts and find the words where I last left off…
…'Baby feathers falling from the heavens…
  Celestial secrets from the gods.'
We are never alone.

October 18, 2000, Barcelona
"What do you want Pauline?"

Just the way you say it dissolves me inside. We both respect the fact that we only have now. Our lives these thirty years have been only within the now. Now we are together, now we are not. Yet when I reach for the pen and begin to sketch, instead of answer, for fear that the spoken word will hurt me again, you persist and I know that it is I who must speak of desires; it has always been I.

Now as we stand on this threshold of hope I find it hard to breathe, to say the words, "I love you Javier." I take your hands in mine "I have always loved you." Even when there were others in my life, there was always you somewhere deep inside, our secret hiding.

It is you that speak now. "We have always loved each other from the very beginning."

~ *And So We Heal* ~

My mind races back to our youth, when yes, I knew it in a moment and yet life did keep us separate all these years.

How beautiful to think that we could hold such love for each other across the distance.

"I want... I want..." The words know that they must be spoken... but I become breathless when I try to speak.

Being with you this last week, observing how you are, your gentle calmness, brings me peace. I am content just to be...in the moment with you. Looking deep into your eyes, a reflection of truth surfaces to meet my own.

"I want us to be together somehow", I say, "to make something together."

But could we have such a reality now that we stand upon this threshold where 'life' hangs by a thread almost?

Inside my heart the words form silently...
Yes I want!
I want ...I want...
I want to melt into your everyday in this way.
Simply to love and be loved.

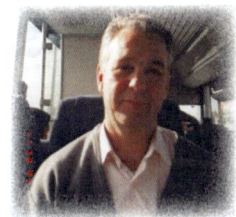

October 27, 2000, UK

I left Barcelona Saturday almost one week ago. Here I am back at my mother's house, talking to you in my diary...As we drove to the airport there was a truck ahead of us filled with white feathers that tumbled out upon us like a snowstorm...'celestial feathers'-I knew that all would be well.

The image of you walking across the airport as I prepared to board my flight will be as clear to me forever, as the image of you at eighteen underneath my window in Ibiza. How the years have danced through our lives and now this enchanted story seems to be giving us a blank page full of possibilities.

~ And So We Heal ~

I spent a few days in London in a cloud almost, waiting for your operation to be completed. It all seemed to happen so fast in retrospect. When you got the hospital appointment my flight was already arranged and fate had played its part...Somehow it was important for us to separate as we had done so very often over the last thirty years. I knew I had to be strong for both of us, knowing somehow that this was not goodbye.

Within the realm of patience and grace, everything is possible.

On the day of your operation I awoke twice, 3.33am and later at 4.44am...knowing we were blessed, a force of angels by our side. At 8.30am when I knew your operation was underway, I felt myself not present anywhere really only inside a dream where I could be with you.

Reality to an observer would see me going to Cleopatra's Needle, sitting there trying to harness energy for you, until through the cloudy skies of London came the bright light of the sun.

Later, still in a reverie I boarded the bus that travelled north away from the crowds in London. Closing my eyes I could truly feel my spirit with you, trying to determine when the operation would be finished, trying to keep balanced and calm but at times feeling extraordinary light and power welling up inside me and

44

~ And So We Heal ~

shooting joy out to you. I put my hand inside my sweater and placed it on my own heart to steady the rhythm. I feel that I was part of a rainbow today and all the colours of your paintings came alive for me to play with. Around 5.55pm I felt perhaps the operation was over. Your sister Marta called me to let me know that everything went well and that you had awoken asking questions, as always.

I've been organizing things, painting, and reading the letters you had saved. So many times I feel myself calling out your name, re-connecting to the sweetness that we two have between us.

My quietness can hear your heart pumping. It can see and feel a great healthy pinkness pumping through you.

October 28, 2000, UK

You phoned last night from the hospital. All that I could say and feel was "Oh my God! Oh my God!" Just to hear your voice, as weak as it was, gave me the energy I need.

Yesterday, I sat on the bus daydreaming, watching the clouds roll through the skies, feeling the sun, somewhere out there, trying to break through. I thought of the many times in the last thirty years when I would come home to England in between the travelling. So many times I would look up into the skies trying to find you. Just to think of you, filled my whole body with an electric joy. Then, as if by co-incidence, a postcard from you would arrive and I knew that you were thinking of me as well.

Part of me has waited always for time with you. I shall try to breathe slowly and calmly and continue painting...where in reality I could run and dance and fly wildly through the skies, so in love am I.

December 31, 2000
Flying...from Liverpool to Barcelona...

Somehow this distance between us has not really existed...
And thinking of you still stirs the ancient echoes of my soul.

~ And So We Heal ~

I trust it to guide us through the 'now'
I am flying now to be with you
To enter… into the New Year 2001 together.

I feel that together we can create something… Some wonderful thing…

January 2, 2001, Barcelona

What I remember of these last hours that have bridged one century to another is a strange ethereal world in which I was embraced by the 'Beloved'.

The smile of your face, your voice… your touch…
Every part of you next to me.
A kiss, long imagined, thrills some eternal force
filling my senses, moving my heart.
I do believe that we have found a way through the portal
back to the future somehow…
where each of us holds a part of the other,
where everything seems new and yet familiar.

I have been here before.

We are constantly told that this kind of reality cannot be sustained, but surely this realm does have a golden key and by the Grace of God we are allowed access more and more often.

January 16 2001, UK

I've decided that I want to write about our story to inspire others, but there are so many words to sort through that sometimes it becomes overwhelming. It's difficult to make out some of the exact dates on the postcards as they go back to the 1970's…exactly thirty years.

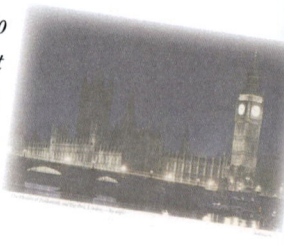

~ *And So We Heal* ~

When I first left the island of Ibiza I am writing steadily in Spanish. Javier had left to live in Holland I remember, and our communication was as friends simple and sweet, basically giving abbreviated accounts of our lives. Unfortunately on the day I left Ibiza my suitcase was stolen with all my letters from Javier. Very little remains.

I begin shuffling through all the 'writings' almost as if I'm shuffling through a deck of Tarot cards, summoning the magic oracle, and there it is - the next clue. I'm drawn into the mystery once again finding little secrets between words and images hidden away for years and years awaiting this time of circumspection.

It is so very true that symbols and words carry powerful energy - *kototama* -the Japanese call It - the soul of a word.

Closing my eyes... I remember moments...

Thank God for that sweet thread of memory winding its way through our lives. You were not like the typical Spanish boy to me... you were blonde even...golden with soft brown eyes, it was your kisses and your embrace as we lay on your bed at the pensión in San Antonio. I can just about remember the location so far back in the recesses of that very young virgin English girl that I was. I remember the passion stirring inside me then, wanting to kiss and kiss and kiss, but nothing more...so afraid to go beyond that which I thought to be 'proper' then. I was a nice girl, and we nice girls must wait until after marriage.

Oh Javier... I do remember that sweetness; it stays with me now even though the other details have diminished through the years. Even then, as now, we were each other's teachers, with Spanish and English.

~ And So We Heal ~

You left for Holland and I, on my journey to Morocco and eventually to Madrid. When I look at what I wrote in the postcards I try to remember where my young mind was…we always signed our letters…your friend, and kisses…besos…xxx. Once or twice I tried to tell you that I was feeling more than friendship… *"I miss you seriously (kiss)."*

That was about as much as I could let you know. We were so young… We had not even made love…so very naïve…And yet our love and friendship has lasted somehow. It has had a life of its own, and now as I look at its rich tapestry I marvel at the absolute grace of this life…the sheer wonder of it all.

I remember reaching Madrid finally and although not intending to stay, remained with my friend and travelling companion Kathy Axford, due to lack of funds to return to England. But happily Spain was in our blood…and there was plenty of work for foreign girls in the nightclubs and bars. We were a great draw for both the Spanish and American service men who flocked to talk to us over a drink. It was fun most of the time and a great way to learn the language. A time of misspent youth possibly, but an important time of freedom, to be independent, with little responsibility. To live with the sun and warmth of the Spanish people, away from the cold reality of England was such a liberating experience.

~ *And So We Heal* ~

> "And over our heads will float the blue bird, singing of beautiful and impossible things, of things that are lovely and that never happen, of things that are not and that should be."
>
> Oscar Wilde

Finally, our story has caught up to us and it seems as if we are trying to fill in the missing pieces. It all seems so long ago now...but last week, all these years later as this new century 2001 began, you said "What happened, why didn't you write for me to join you, or why didn't you say this or that?"

One clear memory I do have is that as soon as I got to Madrid, I called you at your mother's house in Barcelona, hoping so much that you would be back from Holland.

Oh Javier, I called and called, but I could never find you...

I tried...believe me I tried! It's very clear to me all these years later actually- the last time I tried- It was in a restaurant in Madrid around the Plaza Mayor. I was feeling courageous, having had too much wine, but I remember wanting to be with you so much. I was becoming a woman Javier; I was reaching for you...I wanted it to be you...don't you understand?

The time was not ours then...it was not going to be...Destiny stood waiting- the Americans were about to enter the picture. He was actually from South America...I don't know what it was that made me go with him, but I did...although not without kicking and screaming in the end...All the way down the aisle!

49

~ And So We Heal ~

It's not important. That chapter is almost non-existent in my memory now, except that it was the vessel that served to transport me to America - to a completely new life, one that I had never envisioned really, until the day I arrived in Hollywood, years later. Then it all began to make sense. The journey had transported me to the Hollywood of my dreams, and the pain of those married years was a rite of passage, a price to pay, I suppose.

How much say do we really have in our young lives I wonder?

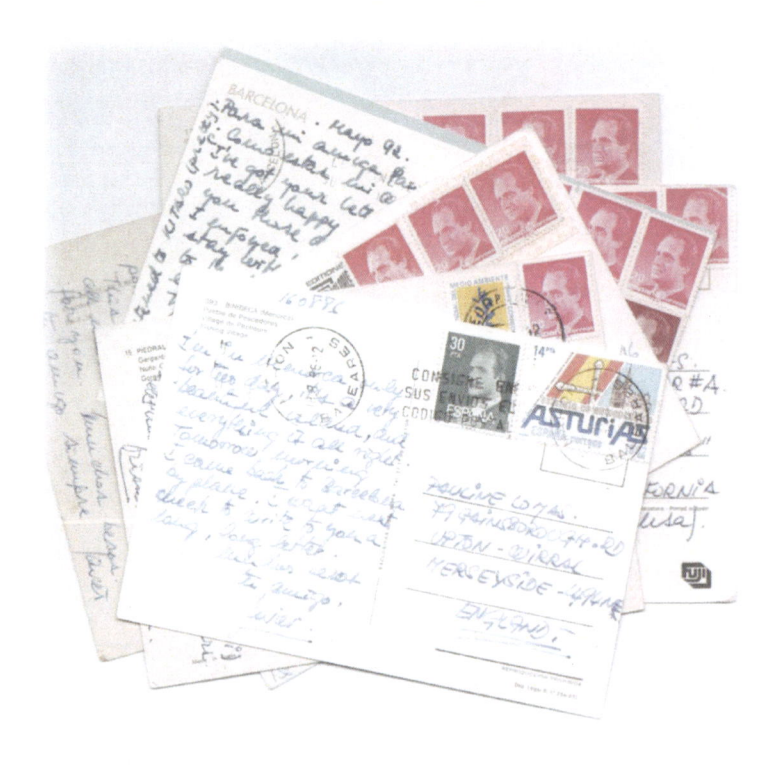

~ And So We Heal ~

The human heart is inhabited by many different longings. In its own voice each one calls to your life. Some longings are easily recognised and the direction in which they call you is clear. Other voices are more difficult to decipher. At different times of your life they whisper to you in unexpected ways. It can take years before you are able to hear where exactly they want to call you.

                                                   John O'Donahue

February 3 2001, UK

The sun shines very brightly today...so rare in England's winter. There is only a short distance between our countries...and no distance between our hearts. I spend my days painting, and writing; trying to advance my business- all to make money to be with you. Nothing is clear...the where and when's have replaced the why's and wherefore's.

I took my sister's little dog Grace for a run in the woods behind my mother's house. There was a crisp chill in the air, but the spring sunshine cast a magical element in the sky and as we approached a favourite spot of my childhood, I was suddenly stopped in my tracks remembering a similar incident many years ago crossing the same field. I wonder if it could be the energy focussed here; as it is after all the ancient site of 'Overchurch,' where the first Runic inscription was found in Cheshire in the 1880's.

I stand rooted to the ground staring at the skies. My eyes well up with tears of joy...for love again...

Nature reminds me that I can have anything I desire now...my dreams are within reach...

~ *And So We Heal* ~

'There is all possibility', the wind whispers.
The doors have opened.
Voices, form words and sentences
spilling over with a desire to stimulate the senses,
erotically seeking to entwine with some fecund warmth,
some other hot breath to comfort what ultimately is so very
fleeting.
Life that is…This glorious bloom of life.

'Follow your heart where love beckons', comes the whisper.
For although the journey may be thread with both roses and thorns;
love and the art of actually feeling for others opens our hearts in ways
that nothing else can…'

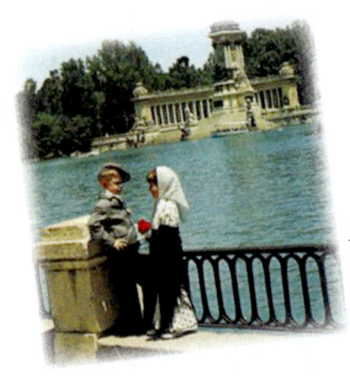

I can…You can…
We can!

As I prepare to sleep now, I ask that I remember my dreams tomorrow…I ask dear Lord for some clear sign to guide me on…I long now for a life with you in Europe.

I am afraid almost to go back to America.

Chapter Four
The Healing Begins

> Last night I dreamed - blessed illusion - that I had a beehive here in my heart, and that the golden bees were making white combs and sweet honey from my old failures.
>
> Antonio Machado

August 2001, California

I had reason to fear returning to America. Something truly terrifying lay waiting in the wings…

Where to begin? After 9.11 perhaps…

Life did make a momentous shift that day, whether we were prepared for it or not. I was in a strange state of mind… even before the twin towers crashed and fell…my world had already been shaken to its core and lay crumbling at my feet. I was back in California, anxiously waiting for my renewed passport in the mail…without it I couldn't return to Europe.

Javier had joined me in California in August, towards the end of my stay, but he was taken ill and had to suddenly return to Spain after only a week. I believe it was a combination of things, especially the medication that he needed to take following his operation, and the excitement of the journey. He wasn't his usual self, and I became distraught with worry, but had no choice but to stay waiting for my passport.

~ *And So We Heal* ~

I didn't realise it at the time but on the flight back to Spain Javier had suffered with a re-occurring migraine that had persisted for days. There was no way he could even begin to talk for any length of time about anything to anybody, let alone to me who had worked herself into such an emotionally unstable state, and with each conversation was wanting confirmation that everything was going to be fine. He had his own insecurities and health issues to deal with, without my needy voice harping on about this and that. It was all too much for him then and silence was a soothing escape. He had chosen that route several times before, surfacing days later with no apologies for his actions except that it was just the way he was. He was from the old school – Bam! – Lock the door, run away – problem solved. Of course he had not had all the years of living in California where 'communication between the sexes' was expected. He had closed the door on me like this in 1992 when we had decided on the abortion. I thought all the pain was locked safely away but I was wrong.

All these years later, knowing so much more about Javier's character I can understand and forgive his behaviour, but at the time there was nothing else to do but bare it and live through this inferno that my life had become.

Now in retrospect I can see that my body was fertile ground for cancer.

I could write little of my true feelings during the days after he left. Looking back at the situation I see that I was trying to maintain the illusion that everything was all right; especially to my friends and family who had all been looking forward to meeting this great 'love of my life'.

August 20, 2001, Los Feliz, California
I have been through sheer hell these last few days. The fire of life - the necessary purification, indeed the necessity of separation within the alchemical process of transformation.

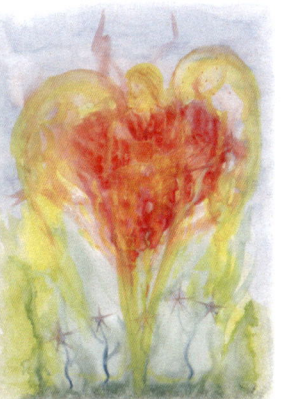

Javier returned to Spain suddenly and when I spoke to him on the phone things did not go well. Fear overcame me as usual...the fear of losing him again is making me so very needy and I feel that I am pushing him away...

I thought that I could never again feel as I do. Large pockets of pain still exist in my psyche and I work hard to free them...push them into the light...

September 10, 2001, Los Feliz California
I've just read that there has been a powerful conjunction of Pluto and Saturn dealing with karma, coming face to face with our fears...the year of the snake- shedding our skin as it were. Driving home tonight I noticed a sign that said 'Torres' meaning 'Towers'...Javier's surname is Infanzón Torre. He is always in my mind, but I cannot reach him. Once again he is refusing to communicate with me...

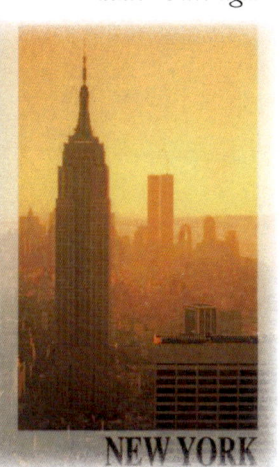

I am afraid that the portal is closing upon us once more.

Who can forget what happened that next day - 9-11!

September 22, 2001, UK
I left Los Angeles one week ago today, following the terrible terrorist attack in America. I am still in a state of shock as is the rest of the world.

~ And So We Heal ~

Several days later following the attack I was able to get one of the first available flights out of America. Whatever it was that was going on with Javier he was refusing to answer my calls.

A few days after he had left I remember having a bad fall on my coccyx causing me to haemorrhage. I was both physically and emotionally ill but trying to pretend that all was well in my life. Returning to England in a state of bewilderment, I cried myself to sleep every night.

It was during this time of deep sadness in my life that I discovered the lump in my breast, and although I tried to think that everything was fine, if I am honest, I knew almost immediately that it wasn't. Nothing prepares you for the horror.

I find these few words in my diary…

October 26, 2001, UK
I went for the results of my mammogram yesterday… The doctor came into the room smiling and so I smiled too.

Then he told me the news… I have breast cancer…

It was exactly one year ago that I prayed for Javier's life as they did the heart by-pass operation…

How can I possibly describe what is happening to me now?

I feel like I am living in another world…it has all happened so quickly that even though I want to write about it, I don't seem to be able to do it justice- perhaps because the 'shock' is still registering in my psyche, and I must work to clear it fully.

~ *And So We Heal* ~

My God, how much braver do I need to be in this life?

Thinking back to that fateful day I remember leaving the doctors and walking out into the parking lot with my sister Deborah. There was this stunned silence and then we both held each other's hand and let out a blood-curdling scream akin to Thelma and Louise just before they drove over the cliff. My immediate instinct was to fight back, and so we drove straight to the supermarket where I bought a mountain of fruit and vegetables. It was winter and I would live on hot nourishing soups, cutting out all dairy, sugar and wheat; embarking on a campaign to detoxify my body. God knows, I had done enough research during Tom's cancer, so I was well informed and absolutely determined to not let this horror get the better of me. First and foremost I needed to repair my immune system. Regardless of whatever treatment a person chooses, it is folly to ignore the vital role that good nutrition and a positive mind plays in healing. This diagnosis was a chance for me to wake-up and take control of my life. My sadness had been eating me alive!

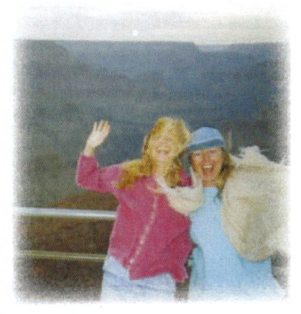

October 28, 2001, UK

Last nights dream was deep and dark:
I was in a jungle facing a wild cat and other dangerous animals. I looked down and saw a lake of water and a rabbit emerging. In the distance I saw a family riding horses and part of me was sad that it wasn't part of my reality. (Perhaps connected to me not being a parent, and to a lifelong wish to have a horse) Then I seemed to fall down a hole, and there was a man next to me and he put his finger in my anus and I screamed, and somehow managed to bite off his finger and spat out a bloody stump! WOW!

This would be the first of many dreams wherein I would be confronted by wild cats… Detoxification would bring the darkness to light …

Slowly I am guided to breathe through this terrible time, where woven through the membrane of my essence, I find an undeniable voice of angelic beings somehow granting me grace…

November 4, 2001, UK
My emotions run the gamut of fear and exhilaration. This is my truth - somehow I feel that I helped create this reality for a reason and now I must 'uncreate' it.

Looking back over the last few months, I remember being elbowed in the breast accidentally early August, then with all the pain connected to Javier returning abruptly to Spain…the fear and confusion was immense…But most of all I remember that I locked the door to my pain and shared it with absolutely no-one. Deep was my sorrow…

This year I have tasted the bitter and the sweet and now as I swallow this most bitter of pills, I strive to keep my spirit in harmony. There is a lot of work ahead of me. I cannot do this alone -

I must call upon the courage and strength that is part of my heritage.

I will work my way through this…into the sunshine of optimum health.

I shall win this fight.
I shall find new joy.
Re-birth for my body, mind and spirit.

~ And So We Heal ~

November 8, 2001, UK

It feels as if I have this canvas in front of me and it is slowly starting to show images…Nothing is certain…I am simply led from one day to the next, trusting that my stamina can withstand.

Every day I feel healthier.

Even though I am detoxifying and my energy level is of course lower, I cannot physically do as much as I used to - but somehow that's ok. God knows I need the rest. Autumn is here and with the winter setting in I need to conserve my energy to focus on the healing.

I've just returned from the Wirral Holistic Cancer Care Center (since moved - see appendix) at St. Catherine's, Birkenhead - the hospital where I was born almost fifty years ago. By some amazing stroke of luck I can actually receive therapeutic cancer care right here on my own doorstep and it's all by donation.

What a strange journey this is…How fragile is life, and how blessed are the gentle healers along the way. Carol, one of the nurses listens to my story and offers compassionate strength and I receive the first of my acupuncture treatments from a wonderful spirit- Beth. She lights up the room and the treatment left me with a wonderful warmth and radiance, and I have maintained my energy level.

I am trying to listen to my own body's needs at present. This morning I awoke with a familiar dullness that appears to be connected to a physical sensation that arises through my body like a wave almost. It's on a cellular level. I feel that healing is at play…the body ridding itself of the toxins.

My dreams are as always very informative:
Last night's found me with a group of people in some sort of mini-bus on our way to the 'spiritual world'. We were laughing and talking about how wonderful this experience was. There was a warm sensation of being loved, but there were no recognizable faces. A message was whispered to me and I in turn informed the others, "Hey everyone...we've got one more day!" It all felt so real....

~ And So We Heal ~

Suddenly I am back in the world of healing and caring for the needy, but this time it is I that need healing.

There had been a period of ten or so years from 1983 in which I was actively involved in helping others through my healing practice of 'Jyorei'. A year spent at Misono, a sacred retreat in the mountains of Japan had instilled in me a sense of service to humanity forging a new direction away from my career in Hollywood at the time. I remember it was during the beginning of the Aids epidemic, and the song *We are the world*' was everywhere. Louise L. Hays had a weekly open healing gathering and we would give Jyorei, often to the many people dying of aids. Helping others to heal had become such a large part of who I am, and this cancer diagnosis was a chance now for me to embody the role of 'wounded healer'.

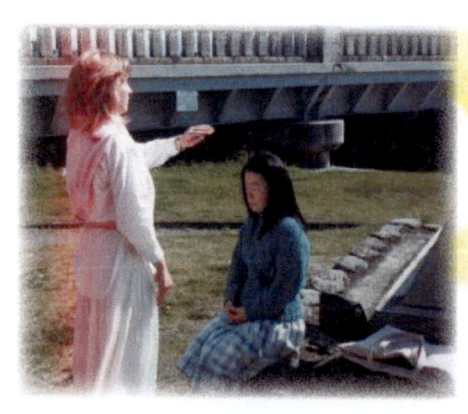

I AM THAT I AM
*I give gratitude
for somehow finding my way
back to the place where I was born,
completing a circle of fifty years,
Trusting all that comes to me now
In*
DIVINE LIGHT AND LOVE

~ *And So We Heal* ~

November 9, 2001, UK

For the past three days I have been using the 'Sacred Path Medicine' cards by Jamie Sams. They are a favourite oracle of mine.

There are forty-four cards in the pack and I shuffle them very well, and each time to my amazement I pick the same card - 28 – 'Medicine Bundle'- allies and support. Now, as I prepare to sleep, the cards accidentally fall around my feet, so I gather them up and as a test I shuffle and pick one. Sure enough, I get it again.

> MEDICINE BUNDLE - Allies and support
> Symbols of connections with allies of the earth.
> Medicines to heal us and give us re-birth.
> Talents to honour, abilities to praise.
> Strength and compassion guide our medicine ways
> The wisdom of the ancestors and allies is supporting
> your present path and should be recognised as
> blessings from your medicine helpers.
> You are not alone.
> Return the favour by supporting others.

November 10, 2001, UK

The 'Champion' juicer arrived today, on loan from the 'Debra Stappard Trust'. Thank God for this, as I could never afford one myself. I'll be able to start some serious carrot juicing three times a day at least.

I've also made the ESSIAC herb tea that I used to brew for Tom, based on the old Indian recipe given to Canadian nurse Renee Caisse, who was well renowned for helping to heal much cancer in her lifetime.

Rene Caisse was born in 1888, one of a catholic family of eleven children and died in 1978. In 1922, she was head nurse at an hospitan in Haileybury, Ontario, Canada. One evening, she noticed that one of the patients that she tended had an oddly scarred breast and asked the elderly woman how it had happened.

~ *And So We Heal* ~

The woman told Rene that over 20 years earlier, she had travelled from England to join her prospector husband in Northern Ontario. Soon after her arrival, a hardened mass appeared on her breast. The area in which they were camping was inhabited by a Native American tribe called the Ojibwe and one of the Indians whom they had befriended was an old Indian medicine man. When he was made aware of her condition, he offered to help heal her and offered her a tea which was a 'holy drink that would purify her body and place it back in balance with the great spirit'. The woman was grafteful for his concern and whilst respecting the Indian's own beliefs, decided to return to Toronto for orthodox diagnosis and treatment.

She was shocked to be told that she had cancer and that the breast would need to be removed immediately. The woman was reluctant to have this operation because a close friend of hers had died recently after a radical mastectomy. She decided to return to the Ojibwe medicine man and take him up on his offer. He gave a tea to drink twice a day until her body was back in balance and showed her how to make the tea on her own. When Rene Caisse met the woman more than 20 years later, her breast was scarred but not cancerous. Rene asked the patient for the recipe for the tea. Her thought was that if she should ever develop cancer, she would gather the necessary herbs and brew the tea for herself. Two years later, Rene used the tea to treat her favourite aunt who had been diagnosed as having terminal cancer of the stomach and liver. She asked permission of her doctor, Dr. Fisher, who reluctantly agreed as he could do nothing further. In two months, her aunt got better. She lived for another 20 years. Rene and Dr. Fisher decided to try treating other patients diagnosed as having terminal cancer. They too showed improvements when treated with the herbal tea and the word spread. Renee Caisse never charged for her treatment, she existed purely on donations. Over the years, news of her work spread and so began many years of harassment and persecution by the Canadian Ministry of Health and Welfare. The story of her work and her struggles with the authorities was told throughout the country in newspapers and by word of mouth and eventually, in 1937, The Royal Cancer Commission conducted hearings about Essiac. In 1938, fifty five thousand signatures were collected on a petition presented to the Canadian Parliament in a move to legalise the use of Essiac. It failed to be approved as an officially sanctioned cure for cancer by three votes.

The smell of the herbs brewing on the stove brings back good memories. I so look forward to drinking it each day - and instinctively know that it will be of utmost importance to keep my system alkaline.

I am grateful that my willpower is so keen and disciplined with all that I am ingesting for optimum health.

A typical day is:

1/3 litre of sun mushroom tea upon rising
Essiac tea, apple juice and E3 live blue-green algae, bowl of fruit - apples, kiwi, berries; banana with living energy sprouted powder and soaked flaxseeds, oatmeal, lots of red-clover tea, lots of assorted supplements

Lunch: *More juice, a hearty vegetable soup with lots of cayenne, ginger, and seaweed, brown rice or other grains*

Dinner: *More juice, soup, steamed vegetables...Lots of herbal tea*

Bedtime: *Essiac tea*

I've cut out all bread, sweets, dairy, caffeine, and try to drink lots of water.

(Slowly I would be lead to whatever nutrients I could afford. There is no end of wonderful natural products that enhance our immune system.)

~ And So We Heal ~

> If a patient can learn to promote a healing from within, that is the cure for cancer...
>
> Deepak Chopra

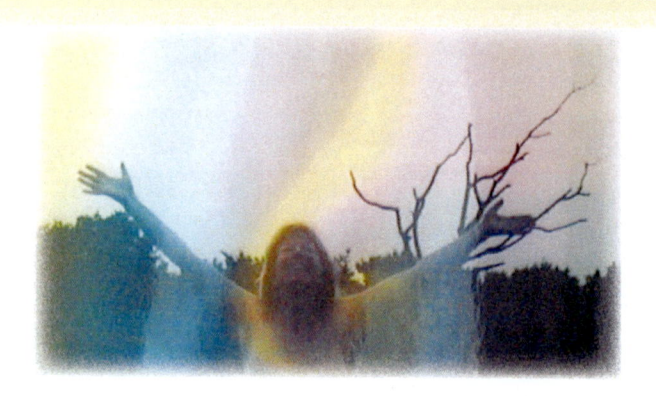

November 13, 2001, UK

It's quite unbelievable how well my body is feeling these days... I am hardly affected by heavy thoughts and am out walking most days... breathing deeply to oxygenate my system. The weather is changing and winter is definitely upon us but the sun is shining most days. I walk my sister's dog Grace, a lot and find quiet places to sit and draw down the sun's energy.

Today as I sat on a park bench meditating there was a powerful sword like beam of white light that emerged from the spectrum of colours I could see in my minds eye. Turquoise, pink and violet rays followed through and I made a conscious effort to absorb their magic message into my cells.

How blessed is this time with nature. How lucky I am.
After the horror of the past few weeks I feel that my body is coming in to balance. I know that it is so much to do with the nutrition, the herbs and the understanding and acceptance of the healing power of

~ And So We Heal ~

> Nature can teach us everything
> Mokichi Okada

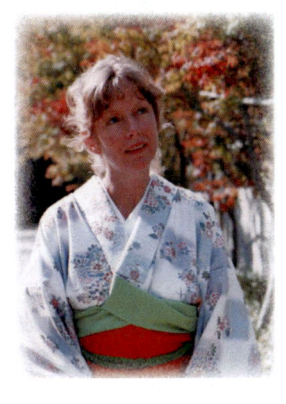

Today in the park the leaves were so colourful - autumn gold's, greens, reds and browns...and then an infusion of vibrant neon, lime-green that came to catch my eye. I soak it in; pull it way down into the hidden recesses of my psyche.

Later, I find the light again in the living room as it catches the reflection of a hanging crystal in the window. It seems to be following me, reminding me of its gift...

I had been having problems with my eyesight so it was time to take action. I was dragging my feet but my mother kept insisting that a doctor look at the scaly red patch that keeps flaring up in the corner of my eyelid. Little did she know that I had bigger fish to fry but finally I take her advice.

November 15, 2001, UK

It's been a long day, beginning with the eye clinic. Thankfully, there is no sign of glaucoma, but the irritating rodent ulcer near the corner of my eye needs to be removed. I've known it for some time. So I will have a scar there...big deal! In the light of what has hammered me lately it hardly seems significant anymore. The vanity of it all died long ago in Hollywood I hope.

I embrace this new life now with the truth of all that I am, as an observer almost, watching life unfold with unbelievable grace.

I have more clarity and less fear.

~ And So We Heal ~

November 16, 2001, UK

Now as I find myself putting words on paper again I unearth all sorts of old memories from Hollywood. They float in as a dream but the reality is that they were my life for a long time. It's only natural I suppose.

The spirit of Tom, my old love is here making me laugh. The words "Trust me", take me back to the hospital room where he lay dying. They were the last words he said to me when I told him I was afraid that his family would not let me see him once they took him home - I was right...they never did.

All these years later I realise how well that pain has healed.

(Excerpt from *"Bridges, a Memoir of Love"*)
'...I knew that Thomas was filled with fear, as so many of us are. I also knew that he was not the only one that had to move beyond it. I've learned so much about fear, this past year—my own especially. My fear of losing love again. Also my fear of death—this was a new one to me. I think I somehow had to climb inside the skin of death to feel it for myself...not just imagine it. There came a series of waking dreams, nightmares, and anxiety attacks when I felt for the first time my own mortality. I faced the unknown void of what it meant to be no longer alive. My own belief in the eternal life of the spirit was of no great comfort to me in those moments...they were my "dark nights of the soul." Working my way through this darkness, I came upon what is perhaps the greatest fear for me - the fear of not achieving my ultimate purpose in life...my mission. It had been a dream of mine forever it seems, to use my talent as an actress to get into the skin of great characters whose spirits touched the humanities in some way and inspired hope in people...'

I still feel Tom's presence at times, laughing mostly like we used to do so much. The essence of his goodness still remains. I did love him

~ And So We Heal ~

and I know he loved me. We were good buddies through the last years of his life, and we had so much fun with an old video camera making our own little films, long before DVD and YouTube...

My experiences have all helped me to understand death, and I am not afraid of it any more. I am just another person whose life has been threatened by disease...There are so many of us.

I shuffle the SACRED PATH' Medicine cards and find:

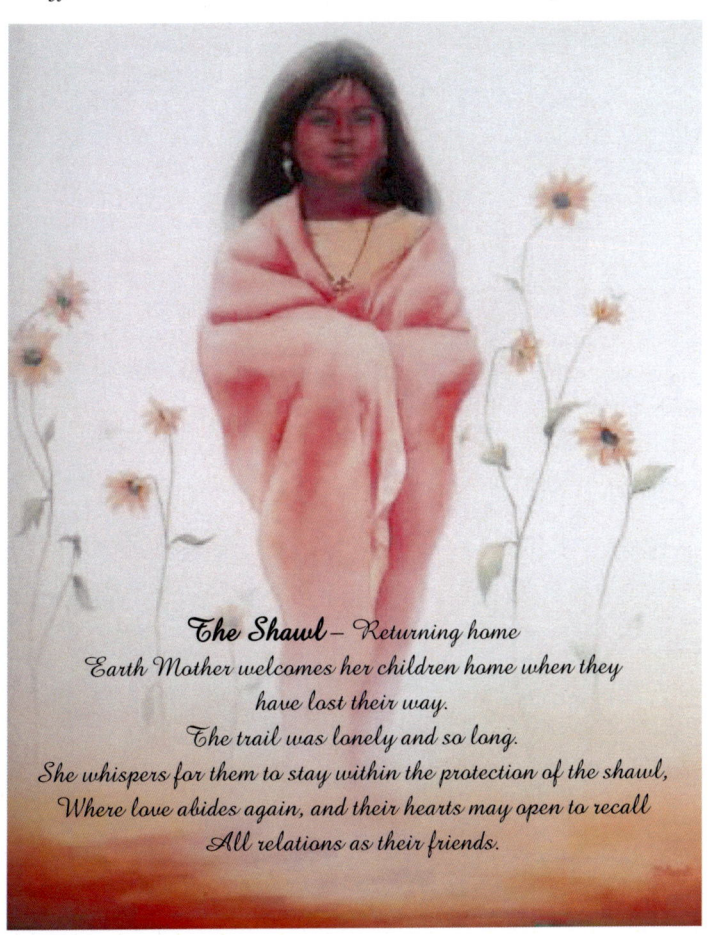

The Shawl – *Returning home*
Earth Mother welcomes her children home when they
have lost their way.
The trail was lonely and so long.
She whispers for them to stay within the protection of the shawl,
Where love abides again, and their hearts may open to recall
All relations as their friends.

~ And So We Heal ~

As my mind and body continued to encourage wellness, I began fostering a sense of gratitude and love for my circumstances.

November 19, 2001, UK

Wherever you are Javier…Please know that I only send you love and forgiveness.

This too shall pass and we shall not lose the thread - that which remains sacred.

I finally pick up the book 'Eternal Echoes' by John O Donahue, *again. So many, many months have passed since I found true inspiration in its pages. What a treasure…*
"There are no manuals for the construction of the individual you would like to become. You are the only one who can decide this and take up the lifetime of work that it demands. This is such a wonderful privilege and such an exciting adventure. To grow into the person that your deepest longing desires is a great blessing. If you can find a creative harmony between your soul and your life, you will have found something infinitely precious. You may not be able to do much about the great problems of the world or change the situation you are in, but if you can awaken the eternal beauty and light of your soul, then you will bring light wherever you go.

The gift of life is given to us for ourselves and also to bring peace, courage and compassion to others."

I am finally feeling free again. All this 'purification' IS a gift after all…

How determined we must be to live!!!

~ *And So We Heal* ~

And so it is I choose to!

Deepak Chopra on Quantum Healing:
Researchers on spontaneous cures of cancer in the USA and Japan have shown that just before the cure appears almost every patient experiences a dramatic shift in awareness. He knows that he will be healed, and he feels that the force responsible is inside himself but not limited to him - it extends beyond his personal boundaries, throughout all of nature. Suddenly he feels "I am not limited to my body. All that exists around me is part of myself". At that moment such patients apparently jump to a new level of consciousness that prohibits the existence of cancer. Then the cancer cells disappear, literally overnight in some cases, or at the very least stabilize without damaging the body further...

Quantum Healing moves away from external, high-tech methods, toward the deepest core of the mind-body system.

This core is where the healing begins. To go there and learn to promote the healing response, you must get past all the grosser levels of the body-cells, tissues, organs, and systems-and arrive at the junction point between mind and matter- the point where consciousness actually starts to have an effect.

November 22, 2001, UK

Each day I uncover another veil to the wounds that I must flush with light. Glimpses of old hurts filter through with this detoxification of my body...the issue of abortion, not having the child with Javier.
I recognise that as a wound still...I must seek to heal it completely.

I remember the voice of my dear wise friend Margaret Maguire - since passed on. Diabetes had left her blind, but any suffering was bathed in the light that shone through her spirit. I would go regularly to give her Jyorei, and we spent many hours together with words of wisdom gleaned upon her path.

"Some spirits are merely touching upon life...not staying...Such

~ And So We Heal ~

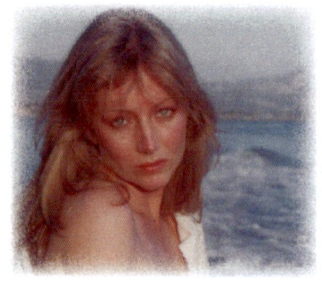

was that inside your body", she said, one day when I sat with her through her dialysis treatment with tears streaming down my cheeks, feeling forlorn about the struggles in my life.

I need to really embrace the pain once and for all and let it disappear from my cellular body.

My love for Javier is such that it shall always be. It is unconditional. But now I must release the expectation and the longing.

I am reminded of a lovely dream two days ago:
I awoke in a small room with Robert Redford. It seems we'd been sharing bunk beds. I asked him about work as an art teacher, referring to a past episode in my life I suppose, when I went to his Sundance Institute selling my art, 'Chalices of Light' The look he gave me contained so much love and understanding. Oh," he said, " I didn't know you would be interested in that."...Or words to that effect...

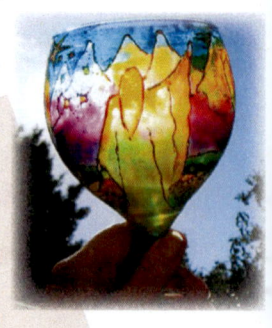

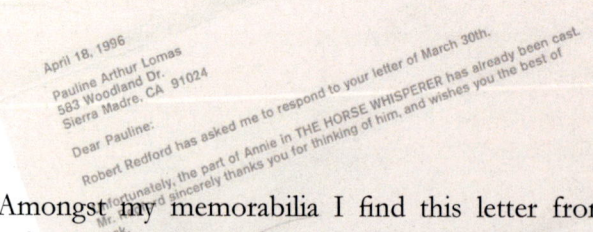

April 18, 1996
Pauline Arthur Lomas
583 Woodland Dr.
Sierra Madre, CA 91024

Dear Pauline:
Robert Redford has asked me to respond to your letter of March 30th. Mr. Redford has asked me the part of Annie in THE HORSE WHISPERER has already been cast. Unfortunately, the part of Annie in THE HORSE WHISPERER has already been cast. He sincerely thanks you for thinking of him, and wishes you the best of luck.
Best,
Vanessa McC...

Amongst my memorabilia I find this letter from him in reference to my wanting to audition for the lead role in his film, 'The Horse Whisperer' He couldn't have known how very much I had wanted it then. It was probably the last film I ever aspired to work on. Destiny again conspiring otherwise.

I have met and worked with many famous people over the

~ And So We Heal ~

years, and often have dreams where they appear to me, so it's not that unusual that I should have these experiences and they help me realise that giving up my 'Hollywood dream' has never really been acknowledged properly inside my psyche, and I remember being highly ambitious at that time…

I do wonder about this. Perhaps I have some cellular clearing to do in that area. I often think of other women I met there and how I always wanted to inspire others through my work, never once imagining that I would have to play this role of 'wounded healer', in order to do so.

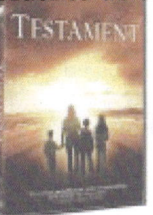

'Bugsy'- I finally got to act with Warren Beatty. As a teenager I remember falling madly in love with him in 'Bonnie and Clyde'.

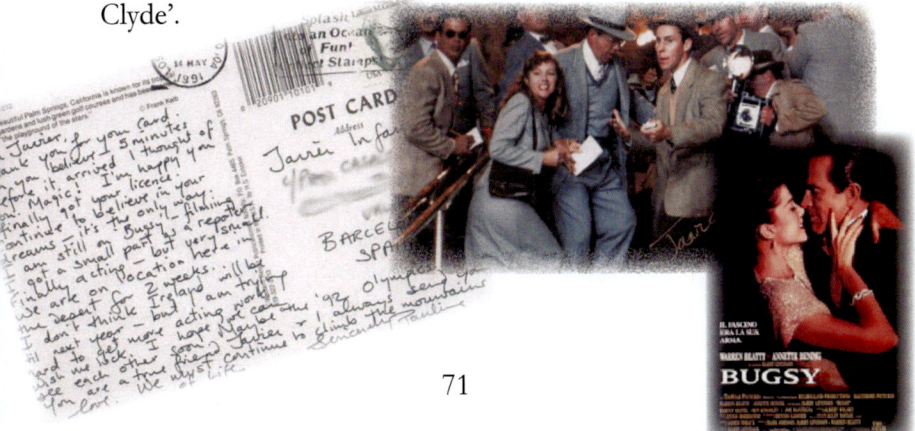

Chapter Five

The Path to Andalucia

November 26, 2001, UK
I shuffle the Sacred Path Medicine cards:

> Warbonnet – Time to advance...
> Do not waste energy on going backwards or staying in the doldrums.
> You are now able to move to the next step on the sacred path. Like a war bonnet chief you have earned the right to learn the next set of life's mysteries. Take your medicine bundle and all of the strengths it represents and charge forward. The advance can be on any level. Your spiritual, physical, mental, and emotional healings are understood through life's experiences. You can now approach your destiny with every feather you have earned marking your past victories and see the destiny you have chosen emerging before you.

Your medicine is strong and will allow the advancement you need at this time

I awake at 3.30 am and prepare to leave for Liverpool Airport.
It is 4.44 by the car clock. Quite a surreal morning to say the least - still and crisp, with a sky of early dawn and the brightest star shining down. My Sister Debbie drove me to the airport - hardly any traffic and the flight was on time.
During the ascent I visualize profound healing...

~ And So We Heal ~

I am leaving for Spain.

And suddenly it seems... am touching down in Malaga.
Ruth Fellner, the owner of the village retreat where I have rented an apartment is there to pick me up. She is sweet and gracious and very compassionate about my 'lump' as I refer to it.
We stop by to pick up some organic produce and after a brisk walk along the sea front we are back in her 4-wheel drive winding up, inland, over mountainous terrain to the tiny town of 'Los Ventorros', near Comares, an old Moorish mountaintop stronghold...It's all so very magical.
I allow my spirit to breathe in my new home...
'El duende' is Ruth's wonderful Oasis in the middle of the desert, a veritable bazaar. Colours are everywhere, every hue imaginable, with rich handicrafts, rugs, pots, lamps, clothes, all manner of delights, and a kitchen full of healthy fare. A familiar magic warms my soul as I am led upstairs to my little abode where a simple Moroccan design invites, and walls of bright yellowy orange envelop me.
I am left alone now to settle...Alone in the middle of unfamiliar terrain...alone with my thoughts...I turn to sadness...
In the sanctuary of my new home, tears come pouring out again as I face what is really bothering me: the fact that Javier still refuses to communicate with me. The tears are insistent...I let them come, all a part of this strange journey.
Slowly I manage to push my sorrowful soul through it, and as the tears subside,

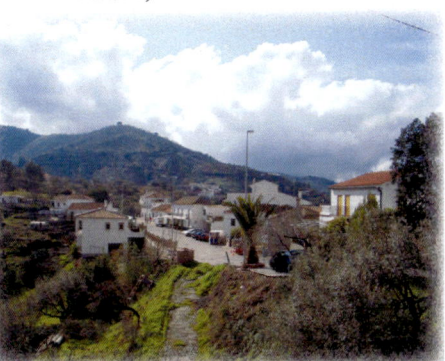

I find grace on the other side.

~ And So We Heal ~

It is going to be all right.

I can be alone. I am tired, that's all. I must close my eyes now and rest. Curled up in the huge king size bed I find calm. The day was still light outside, but I could not venture into it yet. My body sunk below the comfortable quilt and the whole room was aglow in yellow.

Tears spilled again as I cried…But they weren't just for me now… This was so much more - I cried for all the loneliness that people feel.

I try hard not to spend too much time within the so-called negative aspects of my illness. I can hardly bring myself to say the words… 'Breast Cancer'. Is that what I've really got?

The truth is; the reality of it just refuses to register in my psyche. I feel this is to be the key to my well being.

I'm currently reading 'Anatomy of the Spirit', by Caroline Myss. *Powerful information; as with all the books that come to me now:*

THE SECOND CHAKRA- the power of relationships. Located in the lower abdomen- navel area. Energy Connection to the physical body includes the sexual organs. Energy connection to the emotional /mental body resonates to our need for relationships with others, and our need to control the dynamics of our physical environment. Illnesses that originate in this energy centre are activated by the fear of losing control…e.g. ovarian cancer, fibroids resulting from 2nd chakra creative energy that was not birthed…

I am definitely carrying around a lot of broken dreams that were never birthed.

SEFIROT/SACRAMENT CONNECTION

Aligned to the' sefirah of Yod', which represents the phallus, the male energy of pro-creation. This partnership chakra also holds the energy of the 'covenant'. This procreative energy is both biological and spiritual: we desire to create children, and to bring our creative ideas into physical form, which is as crucial to our physical health as to our spiritual health. The sacrament of communion resonates to the energy of this chakra and symbolizes bonds we form with others. Communions of many types are symbolised by the act of sharing bread together.

I know the key to my healing lies within the relationship between Javier and me. I think back to the fall I had on my coccyx, just after Javier had essentially 'abandoned' me in California, and also to the strange dream of being penetrated in the anus, and spitting out the 'bloody stump'- could that have been the root of the tumour perhaps, or was it all just lying in incubation after Tom's death, another 'abandonment', or violation of trust, if you will?

And what of all the broken Hollywood dreams?

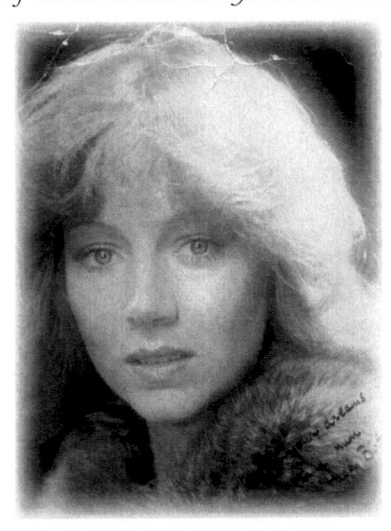

~ And So We Heal ~

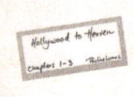

HOLLYWOOD TO HEAVEN

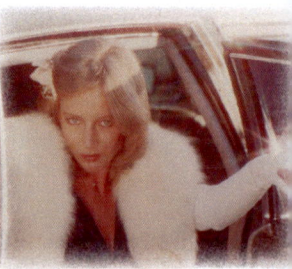

Chapter 1

The words "Second Team on the Set" didn't usually need to be repeated before Jennifer Manning appeared as if spirited by magic onto the required mark to rehearse the shot. But just lately nothing seemed to be going right for Jenny. Her brightness needed polishing and even eternal optomism seemed to be fighting a losing battle. The mirror of time was already reflecting hints of the vacancy and indifference associated with the myriads of disillusioned young hopefuls in search of Hollywood's dream -- a dream that even Hollywood didn't seem to recognize anymore.

Not that Jennifer cared much for its glitter and razzle-dazzle. Thank God those days had passed. Her sights were set on that of being a serious actress for which the 8 years in Hollywood had done their utmost to destroy. Being caught in its net of illusion brought a desperate longing to escape shackled together with a stubborn determination never to give up. But what was blood in Hollywood after all but a man-made substance. She was the last one to realize she was dying.

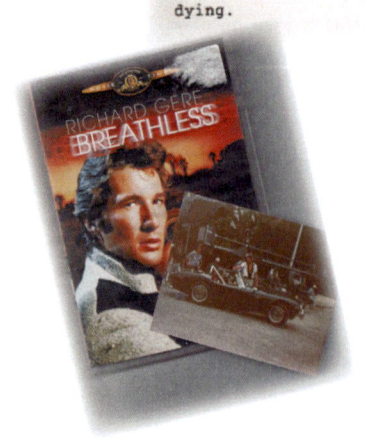

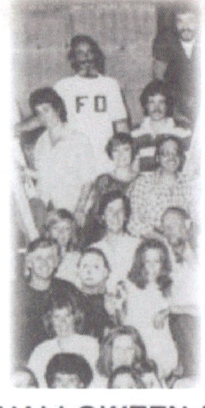

HALLOWEEN II

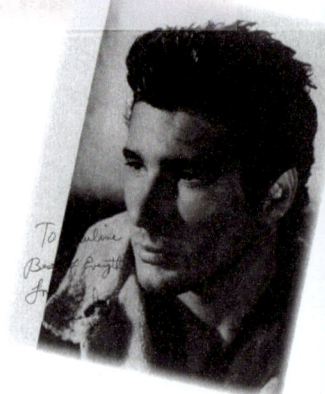

The archetypal energies of the Sefirah of Yesod and the sacrament of communion and the physical energy of the second chakra all symbolise that relationships are essentially spiritual messengers. They bring into our lives and we into theirs revelations about our own strengths and weaknesses. From relationships within the home to those at work to community or political activity, no union is without spiritual value: each helps us grow as individuals. We can more easily see the symbolic value of our relationships when we release our compulsion to judge what and who has value and instead focus on honouring the person and the task with which we are involved. There is an energy working 'behind the scenes', organising when and where we meet people and always at the right time. The spiritual challenge of the 2nd chakra is to learn to interact consciously with others: to form unions with people who support our development and to release relationships that handicap our growth. Physical science recognises 2nd chakra energy as the law of cause and effect, and the law of magnetism. Applied to relationships these laws mean that we generate patterns of energy that attract people who are opposite us in some way, who have something to teach. Nothing is random.

Prior to every relationship we have ever formed, we opened the door with energy that we were generating.

The more conscious we become the more consciously we can utilize the energy of the 2nd chakra.

I am reminded of a strange dream a few nights ago:
Javier and I were seated around a table but not able to talk in depth as a man comes to join us. There appears an image of Jesus with a patch of blood on his robe. He is pointing his finger at someone next to me then vaguely at me. It wasn't too clear, yet I knew it was significant. I somehow feel that these holy images and symbols both in my waking state and dream state are very much a part of a collective psyche.

~ *And So We Heal* ~

Later that same evening, my first night at El Duende, I bought some wonderfully fresh local olive oil and used it to embellish what vegetables I had with some from Ruth's garden. The tomatoes, leek, garlic, chard, seaweed, soybeans and brown rice make a strange mixture, but the key is to be grateful for whatever good food is at hand, and relish the nutrients. It's actually not bad at all, and my little stash of organic dark chocolate and dried apricots finish off the meal, and a hot mug of red clover tea to warm my bones.

Yummm…I'm feeling very cosy in my new little nest high up in the mountains of Andalucia.

The tears are gone now. How magical life can be when we allow ourselves to clear the emotional debris.

November 27, 2001, Andalucia

I awake this morning to the cock crowing, having had a deep night's sleep but waking at various intervals…thinking…recording the various new sounds around me… imagining…always imagining!

You are still here.
Your image will not leave…
'My darling Javier'…
How long it has been for me to write those words…
Here I am in Spain again.
My feet walk upon the same land as you, but I cannot see you,
feel you…
touch you…
Only my thoughts can reach you now…
like so many times before when I did not have you in my world.

***

~ *And So We Heal* ~

Why am I here I ask myself?

"To heal", the voice wastes no time in its echo back to me.
"You must be strong, child.
Allow the nature of this beautiful land to heal your soul.
When the sadness calls, allow the tears to come.
Push them… pull them through with all the dampness of tears
that MUST fall…
Just don't linger there.
Pull yourself out of the depths.
Eat well of all the food that comes to you in goodness and put
yourself upon the path that climbs upwards".

A short while later and I am off to find the historic town of Comares… Downstairs, I stop to chat to Ruth who's busy with the countless tasks around her kingdom. What a magnificent emporium she has created. Everything seems full of health and beauty. Outside, the walls are painted a Moroccan pink and she tells me that is where she bought the paint…in Marrakech. Algeciras is after all only hours away, where there is a boat across to Africa. I think of the two journeys I have made there, and how last year Javier and I had talked about going further south to Essauria.

All my long lost dreams seem a million miles away now…

I try to inhabit the here and now as best I can.

Taking a moment to open up with Ruth comes unexpectedly, and just the speaking of words ushers in more tears. The day will be fragile. Ruth hugs me and gives me Pulsatilla*…homeopathic drops that will calm me when I am adrift on waves of emotion.

*Mostly given to women, the person needing Pulsatilla is sweet-natured, shy, kind and gentle. They are very dependent on others, easily led and may be highly changeable. Public opinion is very important to her and she can feel easily slighted and full of self-pity. They are empathetic people. They tend to be swayed by emotion rather than thought. They are very tearful and will often burst into tears easily, eliciting the reassurance and consolation they need. Pulsatilla people tend to be plump, fair-haired with blue eyes. They can flush or blush easily.

Aha!...Sound familiar?

Walking outside into the noonday light, the village is quiet. Next door, the swish of a slow broom sweeping aside dust...this sweeping of the front steps is so familiar here in Spain- the pace of life so much saner somehow.

I begin my walk up (and I do mean up!) to the town of Comares and soon realise that I am wearing too many clothes for such a venture up the mountain, but I am pleased with my stamina, although I must admit to slight shortness of breath. Taking note of my surroundings, I find layer upon layer of pastel hue stretching out to infinity. The contrasting colours of the olives, the tangerine and orange groves, the white, white houses with terra-cotta roofs all invoke ancient memory.

Were I not still shedding tears, I should be so happy to be here where such beauty abounds... but there is still that part of me that must continue with the purging...and tears fall.

Answers come to my silent questioning...It is all about the pain of lost love...of sacrifice.

Approaching Comares I realise that I am now on a very steep climb... the final ascent to this fairy-tale like village built on the mountaintop. The main plaza area affords a magnificent view of the surrounding mountains. I am reminded of the Moroccan village in the book 'The Alchemist', by Paul Coelho.

Eager to mail the postcard I have written to Javier I am directed to the local post-office; which is to my surprise someone's home. Stepping inside I am greeted by an old man who was obviously midway through lunch…chewing away with crumbs of bread around his mouth. He sells me a stamp for the card and my correspondence gets left on the dining room table with other letters.

Continuing my walk I'm laughing to myself wondering if Javier will ever receive it. Just how often does this high-tech delivery system make its rounds I wonder?

The words I chose to write on the postcard were simple words of friendship, wanting to speak of peaceful things. Hopefully the air between us can be cleared, that is all. My soul needs that.

Later, sitting on a bench I do the chi-gong meditation that a friend has taught me… gathering strong chi energy to infuse my heart and chest area.

It doesn't take me long to make the loop through the village, and chance upon three women gathered outside a small house. English voices echo in the air and I approach to discover that it is actually a centre for natural medicine. A billboard outside offers shiatsu massage, tea and infusions, a variety of healthy fare and English books. Unable to resist this treasure chest of goodies I step inside, and am greeted warmly by a lovely lady, Anna Moore, who invites me to tea. I order a pot of infusion number 2, a digestive tea. While Anna disappears into the kitchen to put the kettle on I browse through the bounty of books. One in particular catches my eye – 'Soul Mates in this Life' - I leaf through it, gleaning sentences here and there, all reminding me that the very nature of soul mate relationship is here to challenge us in ways we need, in order for us to grow.

~ And So We Heal ~

Anna arrives with the tea and sits down with me, eager to hear my story and I, hers. My eyes well up with the usual tears as I open up to this caring stranger, about my lump and my emotional entanglement with Javier. At times I can hardly talk as the emotion rises inside me taking my breath away, especially talking about the pregnancy, and the subsequent termination.

Anna reaches for a deck of cards, an oracle called 'ENLIGHTENMENT', and as instructed I begin to shuffle. A strong sense of truth seems to permeate my being as I close my eyes and pick a card. SACRIFICE- relating to relationships is the card I chose, and as Anna proceeds to read the particular meaning of my choice I accepted the words as they ring true inside my heart…

I had been giving far too much and my lesson now was to be able to receive.

Anna, who is an iridologist, and naturopath, is the first professional to tell me eye to eye that I can heal my disease without surgery. There is something about her manner that is good and strong, and learning a little of her own background and life struggles I am inspired by her story. She had been in a Mormon marriage and a member of the church for most of her life, but four years ago she began to discover her own truth, and felt it necessary to leave the church and her marriage in order to embrace her personal truth. Of course such a decision caused upheaval within her family.

We enjoy a hearty bowl of her home-made soup and fresh bread and feeling much better, with eyes dry, I decide to let her do an iridology session for me as this is one of her many skills. I am fascinated as she explains to me that there are marks on the irises that have recorded past traumas in our lives. Through this ancient practice one can detect the specific weaknesses of the different areas of the body, which are weakened in the process. After pinpointing some of my own weak

~ And So We Heal ~

spots, which make absolute sense to me, she prescribes certain remedies, among them homoeopathic drops for the lymphatic system, and vitamin C powder, of which I'll up my intake to five milligrams a day.

Hours have passed and night is slowly creeping in so Anna offers me a ride back to 'El Duende'. Outside the sky is a rich royal blue and the moon is encircled with a familiar orange glow. It is quite magical. Despite such beauty it is still a little chilly and I am feeling a dip in my energy - it's been a long day with lots of purging.

On the way back we stop at a local goat farm and stepping in to the workshop we are met with a cheery robust woman hands full of a wonderfully enticing cheese. My mouth waters at the thought, but I am quite adamant with my diet at this point and although I forgo this time I know the day will come when I can enjoy it again. Alongside the cheese selection I find some ruddy looking almonds and opt for a bag instead. Driving back down the hill we are confronted by a herd of goats coming home for the night I suspect, funny faces pressing up to the car window. Anna drops me off at 'El Duende' and I hug her gratefully for such a wonderful encounter. I set up an appointment for shiatsu the following Wednesday, and promise to bring some of my 'touchstones' to trade with her.

Inside 'El Duende' I greet Ruth and confirm an aromatherapy session with her friend Sandy the next day. Ruth has made her own home-made tofu today. I purchase a slice, and head upstairs. It is chilly and I am hungry. The tofu mixes well with the leftover soup I heat up... so warming for my soul. Later I enjoy the almonds with dates and mugs of red clover tea, and of course the remainder of the chocolate...

If I'm going to feel guilty about anything it may as well be the chocolate, but it's organic, and somehow I know it too is good for the soul. I thank God for a blessed day...

November 30, 2001, Andalucia

I seem to be adjusting well to the extreme tranquillity of my surroundings. This morning I found myself walking into the neverending mountains simply enjoying the beauty of everything. Each charming white house has a story to tell…the balconies, the windows with their wooden shutters. So many little details seek to remind me that I do not have a dwelling of my own anymore, even though I am truly grateful and feel very comfortable in my mother's house, having spent many years as a youth there… It's like being back in the protection of the womb. I accept that I shall be summoned to wherever it is I need to be to learn the lessons for my healing. This experience is just another magical gem upon my way.

I continue…winding my way upwards pausing here and there to catch my breath and to study the plant life along the road. I breathe deeply of the magnificent air and healing sun; and am reminded of a poem in the book 'Back to Eden' by Jethro Kloss…such a glorious manifesto to health:

'Who is she that goeth forth as the morning - fair as the moon, clear as the sun, And with banner floating above her?
The true healing art.
Whence art thou? - I come from nature.
What art thou? - Herbs, water, food, pure air, sunshine, exercise and rest.
Where art thou going? - On the wings of the morning to the ends of the earth.
What is thy commission? - To every physician and nurse, and whosoever will,
To restore many families, prevent much suffering and premature death, and wipe the tears from many eyes.
Speed on thy flight, thou messenger of health and joy.
Speed on thy flight thou messenger of health and joy.'

~ *And So We Heal* ~

I climb and climb until I find the perfect rock upon which to sit and take the time to meditate. Beginning with the chi-gong exercise again, I'm able to manifest the chi with a remarkable ease.

After focusing on the emotional content of my disease, specifically the 'termination' I was quite able to bring in a strong violet light, and a white light that quite literally pushed into my right breast with such force that I could somehow connect to the pain of the past...As the strong light pierced the wound in my breast I could feel something being pulled out through my body and almost flinging itself out of my left arm with a whoosh... of the chi energy...a wind of elimination rushing through my being.

There are several deaths necessary to erase emotional pain – I accept this as one of them.

It takes great courage to face ones demons...almost like going into battle. Today was a day for release...

Later in the day as I sat writing my diary I could hear the distant voices of the Spanish men in the bar next door. They all sound so familiar...their sound that is...the sounds of Spain are comforting to me.

Another layer to my thoughts comes whispering in...
He is there ...somewhere ...he is always there...
Javier.

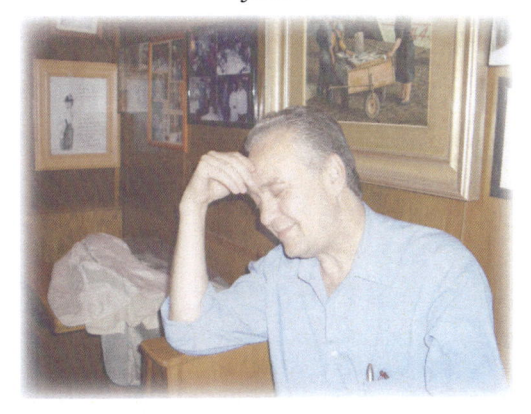

~ And So We Heal ~

I accept this now, not as something to fear any more, as in the fear of being hurt again; as a threat to my recovery…for I shall recover no matter what. It is more a confirmation that I am living in the now… able to observe things and not get caught in the drama of 'us'. Rather an acceptance of the bond of 'us' and that has no limitation.

My dream last night was of Javier and me.
I am playing a drum and he another instrument. Together we struck such a wonderful harmonic resonance...

I have faith that there is much invisible cellular work being done to heal this separation.

December 1, 2001, Andalucia

This morning I went up to the well to fill my water bottle…such a beautiful walk. I so enjoy the challenge of the steep climb now and the chance to open my lungs to breathe in the fresh mountain air. Upon returning I have a hearty breakfast of steaming rice, almonds and apricots with a little soymilk, and after a short rest I am well fortified and ready to ascend into Comares again for the shiatsu treatment with Anna.

Her healing room is very peaceful and the shiatsu is quite amazing. As my body releases its hold I can feel strong violet light flowing through me. After the session Anna tells me that my body was very open to receiving, but that the areas between the throat and the heart, and that around the solar plexus are definitely depleted and in need of energy. It doesn't take much to realise just how out of balance my body has become with all this stress in my life. It all makes absolute sense. I must now by all means attend to this deficiency.

~ And So We Heal ~

I strengthen my heart and heal this with joy

Walking back down the mountain to Los Ventorros I feel full of light and vitality. The twilight fades through dusky lavender to blue and I arrive back at El Duende. Ruth and her daughter, Kayla have gone to England for a few days so I am alone in the house. There is a full moon out tonight, shining round and bright through my window. It's yet another big bowl of vegetable soup for dinner with lots of cayenne and garlic, and steaming brown rice. In anticipation of entering into my 50th year I treat myself to a glass of red wine, and some soul saving dark chocolate.

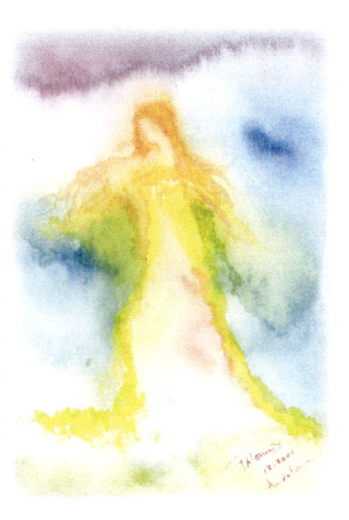

December 2, 2001, Andalucia
The day is finally here…I am 50…

   I have awoken from a drowsy warm sleep to see the sun, blood red and vivid, begin its ascent up over the familiar mountains of Andalucia framed in my window. Light changes rapidly and a spectrum of colours fills the room. I open the birthday cards from family and tears fall…it was my choice to be alone at this time…I did not want all the pressure and stress of the fuss they would inevitably make. It would break my heart…especially since only one of my sisters knows my secret.

   Such a strange day…there's a sadness and apprehension about my life, when really I should be celebrating.

   As I contemplate what to eat in order to give me a boost I hear the sound of the local fish truck arriving, and instinctively I am called… There is not much to choose from but the sardines look appealing and before I know it I am back in my kitchen rustling them up with olive oil and garlic, and just because it's my birthday; a pinch of salt. What a feast!!!

~ *And So We Heal* ~

I look at the clock just as it records 11:11, and I suddenly get the urge to phone Javier. As difficult as it is, I dial his number before fear prevents me. His voice has softened since our last conversation months ago. He tells me he thought my birthday was tomorrow...I am hurt that he has confused the date, but at least the lines of communication are open. I try to talk about what happened between us but he doesn't really want to get into emotional issues...Even explaining my 'need to communicate' just takes us in circles.

He has closed a door on our relationship as he did in the past and for whatever reason I realise that only he holds that key...only he can unlock it. I must retreat...I must.

The time is not right to share the truth about my health. He cannot bear the weight right now. Oh dear God...Why does my life have to be so painful? When I hang up the phone I am momentarily thrown into despair.

My first thought is to fling myself on the bed sobbing, but something stops me...I don't give in to the drama. I shift and move my body instead...reach for the 'rescue remedy' flower essence, and repeat the words... "Stay calm."

A shaft of sunlight calls me to the back window and I stand inside it with my hands in prayer. I am struggling with the words that part of me wants to express...To give Javier up once and for all; even whilst knowing that we still have unfinished business. Part of me wants to scream to the gods...'Take him out of my heart!" and I envision an arrow being shot high into the heavens.

But just as I gather the courage to blast him out of my life forever, I hear voices below and find myself pulling back...not following through...shifting, almost as if I am being led by an external force. I find myself wandering through the house instead, and as if by some divine guidance am led to the bookshelf whereupon I find one of my favourite books, 'The Alchemist' by Paul Coelho.

Opening it up I am met with the words:

~ And So We Heal ~

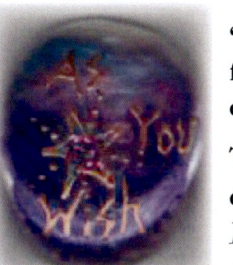

"In order to find the treasure you will have to follow the omens. God has prepared a path for everyone to follow.

There is a force that wants you to realise your destiny."

For the rest of the day I remain in a state of grace about life, and enjoy re-reading 'The Alchemist'. Come evening I call my mother, knowing that she probably wants to wish me a happy birthday.

"Oh…I was going to call you tomorrow, to wish you a happy birthday", she says. Not another one!

"But it's today", I say, frustrated by the fact that nobody seems to be remembering my special day, when in actual fact it is I that has ran off to be alone with the goats wandering the Andalucian countryside.

But she is adamant about this one…

"No it's not", she says with equal frustration. "It's tomorrow!!"

And you know what …she was right. I ran to check the calendar… What an idiot I am…I couldn't stop laughing. Oh that was the biggest laugh ever and what a great gift from the universe…I'd spent the entire day musing the fact that I was now fifty, when in actual fact I was not…still had another day to go.

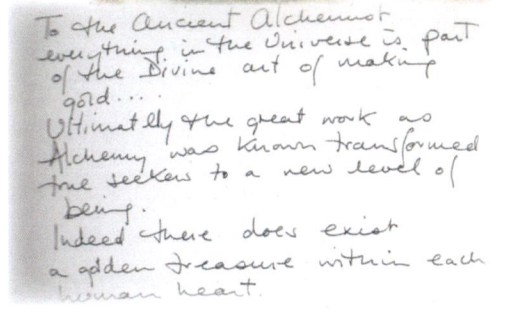

What grand illusion!

Happy, Happy Birthday Pauline!

To the Ancient Alchemist everything in the Universe is part of the Divine art of making gold....
Ultimately the great work as Alchemy was known transformed true seekers to a new level of being.
Indeed there does exist a golden treasure within each human heart.

Chapter Six

Ultreya

I come across this word, 'Ultreya' reading Shirley Maclaine's book, *The Camino*, documenting her sojourn on the 'Camino de Santiago de Compostella', a pilgrimage across northern Spain. I had hoped to make the same journey myself before this little detour.

It means 'MOVING FORWARD WITH COURAGE'

December 12, 2001, UK
*I arrive at the Wirral Holistic Centre as all the 12's hit...**12.12.12**, the twelfth hour of the twelfth day of the twelfth month.*

Beth administers the acupuncture, which takes effect immediately, balancing the hormones, allowing me to drift off with my thoughts...

The sun had shone through the window on my journey here, all so very surreal as it was only yesterday that I was rolling through the mountains of Andalucia, on my way to the airport.

I know I will return to Andalucia one day, but for the moment, there's still lots of work to do...

December 14, 2001, UK
Today I met my new Oncologist, Alison Waghorn at the Linda Mc.Cartney Cancer Clinic in Liverpool. She is very nice, and I was pleased with her ability to be very 'one on one', despite the fact that the waiting room is full to overflowing. Overall the experience was do-able, although the inevitable poking around the breast is never pleasant. She

discovered a swollen lymph node under the right arm, which is not good news of course.

January 10, 2002, UK
England, my family home... How grateful I am for these days...especially through the trials. Dear God...that is when I know with all the faith in the world that I am held by grace.

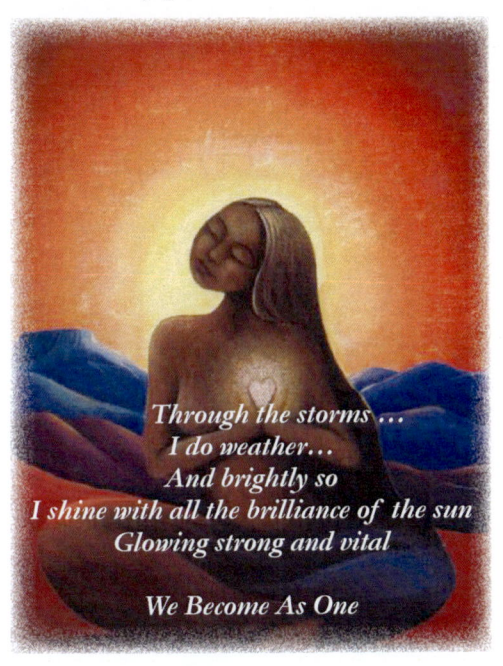

> Through the storms …
> I do weather…
> And brightly so
> I shine with all the brilliance of the sun
> Glowing strong and vital
>
> We Become As One

January 13, 2002, UK
There's a new moon, and I'm recuperating after the minor surgery to remove a basal cell growth on the bridge of my nose near my right eye. I tried to resist the operation without luck and found the whole experience quite awful on many levels. Now, as the scar heals I find myself with an inner gratitude for the experience, and am especially certain now that I made the right choice in electing not to have the surgery on my breast. I feel that I have somehow escaped death.

~ And So We Heal ~

I choose another SACRED PATH MEDICINE *card from the pack:*

Storyteller... (Expansion)
The storytellers of Native America are the guardians of our history and Sacred Traditions...Keeping ancient knowledge alive. This card speaks of expansion on all levels...growth encompassing many new ideas. Feed your personal Fire of Creation. Many lives are influenced by another's story. The wisdom of the storyteller is part of the art of remembering. You are now remembering your personal medicine and how to be your potential.

January 13, 2002, UK

In moments like this I truly feel healed from all of this.
Somewhere within my essence grows this wonderful garden
Fresh, vibrant nature, simple, organic... Full of promise...

January 14, 2002, UK

I get fear coming to play today... How easily it can slip in. I must fight hard to find my balance. Usually when I take twenty minutes or so, to be still, and to glean the many riches that come into my mind, I emerge from the fear with new strength and courage for the journey. Slowing myself down like this I am able to really appreciate the pull of nature, and am beckoned to the back bedroom window - my room as a youth...

Simple nature, pale blue skies...
Earthly green and gold pastel trees,
Shed bare by the presence of winter.
Birds fly back and forth
through the clearing in the woods...
I salute them, honour them; note their colours.
One white ascending, two black descending...
Two white... together... We communicate.
Their voices remind me of healing worlds...
Their wings contain the feathers of my
HOPE

~ And So We Heal ~

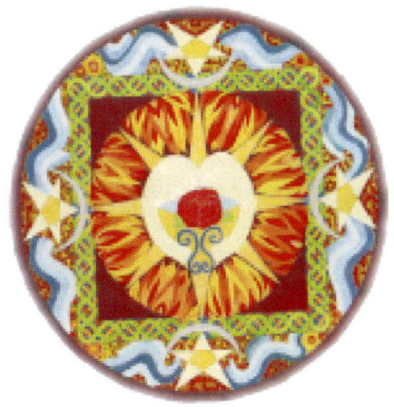

Affirmation:
Today I release love into my body
For I lovingly approve of myself
Love heals my body
Love heals my mind
Love heals my emotions
Love is a healing force

Rosella Longinotti

January 16, 2002, UK

Had my appointment with Dr. Richardson at the Old Swan Homeopathic Centre in Liverpool. What a lovely gentle man. I felt none of the usual trepidation associated with my visits to see doctors.

It helped that he took the time to hear all about me as a person, really listening to what I had to say about my beliefs. It was quite an intense session as I allowed myself to open up about the sadness in my life and my relationship with Javier.

Tears fell as usual around the deep core issues clinging to my being. There seem to be so many broken dreams still stashed away inside my heart.

In about five days, I will receive the Iscador - mistletoe* that I have researched, and then I can begin my series of injections three times a week to find the right dosage.

*Mistletoe was first proposed for the treatment of cancer in 1920 by Rudolph Steiner, an Austrian Swiss physician who founded the Society for Cancer Research to promote mistletoe extracts and anthroposophical medicine.

~ And So We Heal ~

Mistletoe preparations are used to stimulate the immune system, to kill cancer cells, and to help reduce tumor size. It may also help improve the quality of life and survival of some cancer patients, especially those using chemo and radiation, and may help reduce pain and side effects of these treatments. In addition, a German study done by Dr. Ronald Grossarth-Maticek of the Institute for Preventive Medicine in Heidelberg shows that, when used as adjunctive treatment in patients with a variety of cancers, it can increase survival time by as much as 40%.

In animal studies, mistletoe preparations have helped fight some forms of cancer. The best results with Iscador are claimed for its use with solid tumors both before and after surgery and radiation. Given 10 to 14 days before surgery, it is thought to help prevent metastatic spread due to surgery and to promote recovery and it is also used for advanced stage, inoperable solid tumors, especially cancers of the bladder, stomach, intestine, genital organs, and skin. It is also claimed that bone metastases are retarded in some cases. Results appear less promising for inoperable cancers of the breast, lungs and esophagus. It is thought that tumor growth slows or stops, and then gradual regression begins. It is believed that tumor cells are transformed first to a semi-malignant form, then to chronic inflammation and finally to normal tissue.

If money was no object I'd take myself off to one of the many holistic clinics like Lukas Clinic in Germany. (See appendix)

Later I drive with my sister Barbara to the farm in Thurstaston to get organic carrots. Barbara was always under the assumption that my tumour was diagnosed as benign. At the time she herself was undergoing gall-bladder surgery, and I had elected not to worry her. Today however the barriers were down and as we drove through the always-breathtaking countryside, I could not continue with the lie and the truth spilled out. After her initial shock she was of course completely supportive; I just didn't want her to worry, but of course one does…In any case we had a good long hug…and I still elect not to concern my mother and we agree to not tell her.

January 17, 2002, UK
When I went to Arrowe Park hospital to have the stitches removed from the basal cell surgery last week, I found myself offering courage to one of the nurses attending to me. As she was preparing the room she started talking to herself, but loudly enough for me to hear, agitated obviously, but including me as a listener.

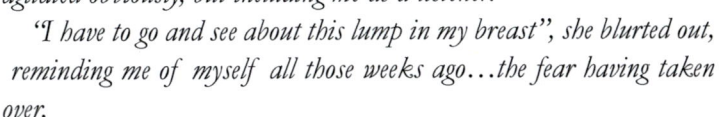

"I have to go and see about this lump in my breast", she blurted out, reminding me of myself all those weeks ago…the fear having taken over.

"I can't sleep, I'm nauseous all the time…I can't eat", she said. I motioned for her to give me her hand, and found myself saying to her very firmly.

"No matter what they tell you…you can handle it!"

Our conversation led us out into the corridor for an intense twenty-minute talk. Luckily I had a pocketful of 'Touchstones'…She picked the word 'Love'.

I reminded her that Love does truly heal and that whatever was happening in her physical body was connected to her emotional body.

In retrospect, I suppose I had 'administered' some kind of supportive care to the very nurse who had actually been assigned to care for me. Some days are like that!

From there I ventured back out into the winter weather. It was actually not too cold and I managed to walk all the way back into Upton to see Alan Hudson the Herbalist. He welcomed me in with a wonderful smile, sat me down, and set off to prepare my 'sun mushrooms'. Singing aloud, his voice echoing through the building, a sad ballad of lost love; the man is a gem...

"Here we go then,' sun mushrooms' it is".

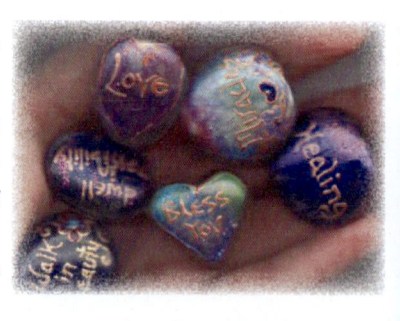

Alan's bright face appears around the door, eager to know how I was doing on the healing journey. I told him that I was gearing up for my Mistletoe injections, and had really missed the mushrooms...

"One thing to remember," he says, "Put the focus on 'getting healthy' ...not...woe is me I've got cancer".

"NEVER LET CANCER OWN YOU!"

Alan's words register strongly on my psyche.

He takes time to relate a story to me of when he had severely burnt his legs after wading in toxic chemicals.

"We're talking to the bone", he says, my face grimacing at the very thought. They rushed him to the hospital, but before he left he packed each leg in a poultice of mallow and some other herbs that draw the toxins out. He refused any antibiotics; and instead had his wife mix him up a prescription of herbs. The doctor said his recovery would take eight weeks. He walked out five days later. Just listening to Alan lifts my spirits.

I give him a pick of the 'Touchstones'. He picks 'Peace', and another one jumps out of the bag - 'the Eye of Horus', an Egyptian symbol meaning 'All is well'.

Leaving Upton, I catch the bus to the 'Wirral Holistic Centre'. The acupuncture I receive there has really been helping my state of mind. I usually meet my friend Jane there and we spend time discussing the various holistic treatments that our research digs up. Jane should have been a biochemist; she really has a brilliant mind and teaches me a lot. I on the other hand have this mountain of faith and a pocket full of touchstones to give away, so hopefully we make a good team, as we inevitably meet and help support others at the clinic who are in some kind of need.

All is well

January 18, 2002, UK

It feels so good to be spending a beautiful winter's day just pottering about, where once upon a time as a child I used to hate Sundays because they were mostly stay at home days, especially during winter. There was the usual big family dinner with roast potatoes and fresh mint from the garden, to have as sauce, with the lamb, or the chicken or roast beef. The tastes return to me now as I take this time to heal. It has been many, many a year since I ate meat, since the early days in Hollywood really. For the moment, it's still much of the same...raw broccoli salad, with grated beets, carrot, ginger, garlic, nori seaweed flakes and heaps of flaxseed oil. Following that a big bowl of brown rice. I'm chewing my foods a lot more lately, and really trying to appreciate all foods as they come to me.

When Tom was diagnosed with his melanoma we went on a tour of the many cancer clinics in Mexico. Again, they were not cheap although I was prepared to take out a loan to help Tom, but ultimately he took a different approach. I always maintained that if it was me I'd go for the holistic approach so the Gerson Therapy appealed to me (see appendix), although I could only apply it about fifty percent, as it entails having a fulltime helper to prepare the juices etc. Hopefully I can increase the carrot juicing, at least to three times a day even though it's so very time consuming, and really means that I need to stay around the house to do so. I've started doing daily coffee enemas.

~ *And So We Heal* ~

The coffee enema is, without question, the most unusual part of Gerson's combined regimen, and often evokes astonishment and mirth in persons who have never experienced an enema and who emphatically prefer to drink their coffee. Practitioners and patients who have had experiences with coffee enemas, however, know that they are far more than a means of introducing stimulating caffeine into the bloodstream. From the patient's point of view, the coffee enema means relief from depression, confusion, general nervous tension, many allergy related symptoms and, most importantly, relief from severe pain.

The coffee enema has a very specific purpose: lowering serum toxins. Dr. Peter Lechner, who is currently conducting a trial of the Gerson cancer therapy in the post surgical treatment of liver metastasized colorectal cancers under the aegis of the Landeskrankenhaus of Graz, Austria, reported in 1984 "Coffee enemas have a definite effect on the colon which can be observed with an endoscope. Wattenberg and coworkers were able to prove in 1981 that the palmitic acid found in coffee promotes the activity of glutathione S-transferase and other ligands by many fold times above the norm. It is this enzyme group which is responsible primarily for the conjugation of free electrophile radicals which the gall bladder will then release."

They are indeed a blessing. So too, the lymphatic drainage massages with Helen Jefferson in Chester which are so vital to my programme. I had my third treatment three days ago…it's not for the weak-hearted. There is so much solid flesh clinging to my bones…flesh that will not allow the lymphatic fluids to flow freely. Helen, one of Life's angels, bless her, puts so much passion into her work. An Australian woman who saved her husband's life when they were living in the outback taught her the technique. It is extremely painful at times, but deeply satisfying. I manage to put myself in a trance-like state so as not to experience the reality of it. Following the extensive pummelling of the areas most blocked, I am swathed in hot steaming woollen blankets that induce a good sweat, pulling out all the toxins. It sounds like quite an ordeal,

~ *And So We Heal* ~

but the next day I awaken feeling fantastic, with an extra bounce in my step.

> **I feel with all my heart that I am healed…**
> **that I am whole…**
> **that 'yes'…cancer can be cured.**
> **There is hope…**
> **We can find our way back to health – naturally.**

January 23, 2002, UK

The weather has been beautiful again. I enjoyed time in the park this morning with my sister's dog, Grace. How my life has turned around in these last three months…

> From death to life…
> all such a blessing… all a decision.
> All, so much by the Grace of God.
> I truly feel alive
> Vital and healthy.
> Grateful to be growing again within the soils of my birth.
> Here I learn to appreciate the simpler things…
> The gentler rhythm of life.
> Somehow, everything is provided.
> My fresh juices,
> my light…from the sun…from nature…
> From the love that radiates
> Through
> network of family and friends…
> Through
> all that I love
> and all that loves me.

99

~ And So We Heal ~

January 24, 2002, UK

I think of you Javier...

Yes...so very many times do you come to my mind...and I wonder how you are, and if you are thinking of me. I find some of your old postcards, and they always seem to say," I am thinking of you", or "you are always in my mind".

Just to see your written word fills my heart...touches my essence in sweet ways.

I wonder...
Do you sometimes feel my thoughts brushing up alongside your mind?
Do you follow sometimes?
When I push on through the portal that I have marked,
'US'

I can't remember when exactly it was that Javier began to get back in touch with me, but he did. I had elected not to tell him about my disease when I was first diagnosed. He was still in his reclusive state and I was concerned that it would all be too much for him to bear. It would take months before he finally began to emerge from his cave and ask about my health. I mentioned that I had a lump in my breast, trying to downplay the situation, but he was insistent with his questioning.

"But it's just a lump?" he said, hopefully
I couldn't hold back any longer, as my eyes filled with tears and my voice told him the truth.

"No Javier.... It's cancer."

How I hated having to use that word. I almost never did.

It's all a bit unclear now as I search my memory to try to remember our conversation that day. I do remember telling him that I had decided to follow a natural course of treatment which meant I had to do a lot of soul-searching inside myself to help me release a lot of the emotional pain I was still carrying, He asked me if I blamed him for what had happened. How could I possibly blame anyone least of all him when I loved this man with every fibre of my being. I do remember waking up from a dream one night however saying the words 'F—k you Javier', so there was definitely a release of anger on some level, but for the most part love and gratitude were what I tried to focus on. Honest!

Lo and behold...the portal had opened again.

June 10, 2002, UK
Today I feel the energies connecting us as opposites. The wind is blowing and we have sunshine and rain.

Fresh air blowing through...
Where this morning I began my day slowly,
still in my yesterday, where it was Javier's birthday.
I thought all manner of things...
and in the end when tomorrow came, he was still there.

August 4, 2002, UK
Javier called this afternoon. It's still very difficult for me to talk on the phone when my mother is in the house, since she still thinks the tumour is benign. I sense fear in his voice when he asks me about my health. I suppose I should just say I feel great and not give away any of my own secret fears. But as small as they are; they are still valid, and I do need to talk about my feelings. It's just that with Javier's heart condition, there is only so much he can handle.

~ And So We Heal ~

It's been a particularly rough couple of weeks dealing with my appointments at 'The Linda McCartney Clinic'. I arrived in Liverpool as Queen Elizabeth was meeting Sir Paul McCartney at his exhibition in the Walker Art Gallery. I came in on the bus, surreally floating as it were, through the tunnel, under the River Mersey.

Having just watched a spectacular display of light during the closing ceremony for the Commonwealth Games the night before I am inspired and feel somewhat electrically charged, if you will, for the future.

August 8, 2002, UK

Still in my dream state this morning, when these words came filtering through...
"And man may heal through his own hand."

So few words actually make it to paper these days. I trust that they shall flow through the tapestry that is to be this book. Meanwhile, thank God I still make time to paint, as it is art that truly feeds my soul these days. I can lose myself for hours upon hours lost in a magical world of creativity.

September 3, 2002, UK
Finally get pen to paper, and write...

I search for answers to the small things... one step at a time.

The guidance is still clear, although sometimes I have flashes of immense fear and sadness. They pass increasingly fast, so bearable to say the least.

The last few days I've been absorbing the shock of actually being judged able to work. It seems that because I am treating my condition in as natural and healthy manner as possible, without surgery, radiation and chemotherapy; the recommended, indeed only option of

~ *And So We Heal* ~

NHS treatment available; I am now considered healthy enough to return to work. What they have failed to comprehend is that ALL my time and energy is devoted to restoring my health and shrinking this tumour.

This IS my work.

The fact is I have an egg sized cancerous tumour in my breast, which by their own admission, is life threatening, and yet there is very little choice within the NHS protocol. Either I accept what they have to offer or nothing.

Extensive research is being done on natural cures, and more and more people are finding less invasive ways to heal themselves. It is frustrating to discover so much valuable information that I and others could really benefit from and yet there is no funding available for some truly wonderful alternative treatments of my choice.

I don't want to seem ungrateful, because I do appreciate the value of orthodox medicine, but statistics show that we are no further ahead with the 'cure for cancer'. It's big business all right!

"It is not enough for the physician to do what is necessary, but the patient and their attendants must do their part as well and circumstances must be favourable" Hippocrates

September 4, 2002, UK

Today was my bi-monthly visit to Dr. Richardson my homeopath - such a gentle man. I released some emotions that had been stifled, and expressed my anxiety about my benefit support being withdrawn. The thing is, that as small as it is, it helps cover the costs of the ever increasing list of supplements my body needs, none of which are available on prescription. He assures me that he will write a letter to support my case and, I immediately start to feel more hopeful. It was good to see that I could snap back into the positive.

~ And So We Heal ~

It's funny really stepping back and observing myself. I guess what I'm trying to do is document all this, forcing myself to keep my pen moving, difficult as it is sometimes.

The more that I take deep breaths and affirm to myself
that I can overcome all obstacles to regain my vitality,
the more it is so…

BREATHE DEEPLY!

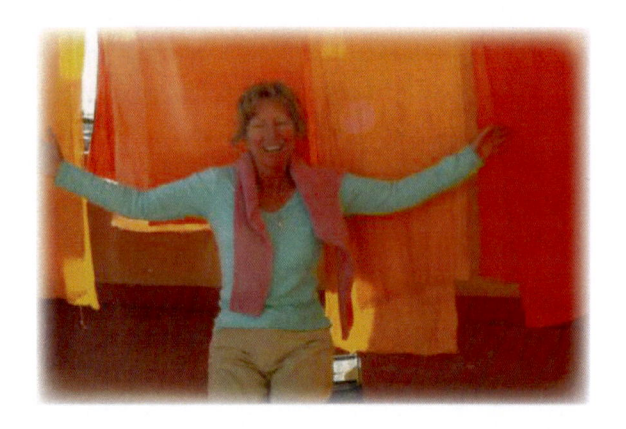

I would like, somehow to be a bridge to new worlds
of medicine.
I shall continue to walk in beauty,
doing my best to uphold the courage
of my convictions and
Heal

~ And So We Heal ~

> Your pain is but the breaking apart of the shell that encloses your understanding.
> Kahlil Gibran

September 5, 2002, UK

I had a dream that Javier and I were cracking open two vials of Mistletoe (Iscador). The glass vial was jagged around the edge of Javier's and he drank the liquid.

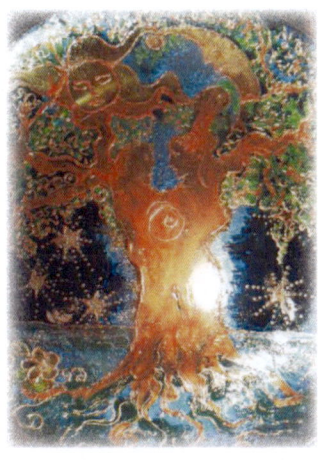

The Druids held that the Mistletoe protected its possessor from all evil, and that the oaks on which it was seen growing were to be respected because of the wonderful cures which they were able to affect with it.

Scandinavian legend has it that Balder the God of peace was slain with an arrow made of Mistletoe. He was restored to life at the request of the other gods and goddesses and Mistletoe was afterwards given into the keeping of the goddess of Love, and it was ordained that everyone who passed under it should receive a kiss to show that the branch had become an emblem of love, and not of hate.

Mistletoe, or Viscum album is a semi-parasitic plant that grows on oaks and other trees in Europe and Asia. Mistletoe is also found in America and Korea, but normally only the European species is used in the treatment of cancer, inflammatory conditions and AIDS. The leaves, twigs, and berries are what is used to make these herbal medicines. Because the medicinal doses are small (it can be poisonous in large doses), many believe it to be "homeopathic," but it isn't. Mistletoe extracts are marketed under several trade names, such as Iscador, Helixor, Eurixor, and Isorel, most of which are available in Europe. Weleda AG manufactures Iscador, which consists of fermented extracts of mistletoe, sometimes combined with trace amounts of silver, copper or mercury.

I've been having annoying little pains in the breast, which I choose to think of as a healing acceleration. I'll be glad to get back on the Iscador tomorrow. I usually have a two-week cycle (every other day) then off for one week. It's interesting to see how it all affects the menstrual cycle. I must remember to do the Castor Oil pack tomorrow that Edgar Cayce* recommends - always quite messy but really soothing and effective.

*Edgar Cayce has been called the father of the modern-day holistic health movement, and his physical readings continue to be studied by physicians to determine it the material given for specific individuals years ago can be used today to help those who suffer from similar conditions. The principles of health and healing in the Edgar Cayce readings are that the balance of body, mind, and soul are so closely intertwined that the dis-ease of any of these three aspects will also affect the other two.

Castor oil is derived from the bean of the Ricinus communis or Palma Christi (palm of Christ) plant, having beautiful large palmate leaves. Through the Cayce readings, it is apparent that the oil of this humble plant is a marvellous source for a multitude of natural remedies. Castor oil is mentioned for use in the form of external oil packs in over 570 health readings. The packs were indicated for use in a wide variety of health situations, from arthritis, to liver and intestinal conditions, to scleroderma. Additionally, castor oil was sometimes recommended for use in massage for various skin disorders, tumours, and breast cancer. Clearly, the beneficial usage of castor oil is wide ranging indeed!

The standard castor oil pack is made from several layers of white wool flannel, folded to about the size of a 10" by 14" rectangle. The white wool flannel is then saturated, but not dripping, with cold-pressed castor oil. In many cases, the oil is warmed before use.

~ And So We Heal ~

November 4, 2002, UK

Tears fall this morning. It began yesterday - this tipping off balance feeling - a few physical symptoms, an eye infection and a growling in the womb, and now this dissolution of tears. But at least I am feeling...

These past weeks I have been unable to put pen to paper, and there is so much to write about.

In September I was once again asked to narrate for the Shumei Taiko Ensemble, Japanese drummers on their European tour through Switzerland, Austria and Germany. It took a lot of effort and courage on my part to make the journey, especially since I have such a complicated health regime every day, but I knew that I would receive a lot of 'Jyorei' and the whole experience was so uplifting and healing in many ways.

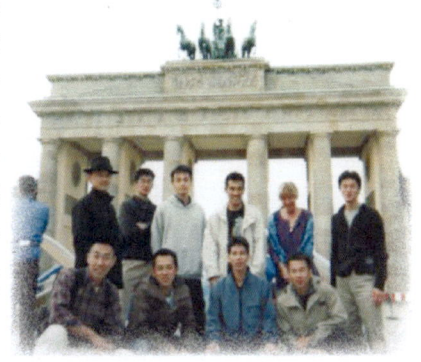

I wrote an article on their performance at The Global Peace Initiative for Women's Religious and Spiritual Leaders in Geneva:

*Excerpt from 'PEACE AMONGST PEOPLE:
I arrive at the rehearsals with the haunting melody of flutes playing 'Hikari', and light breaks through to stir my soul. It is a familiar piece to me now, but this time as I listen, I am aware that the strains of the music stop at the portal of my heart. Where once it opened so easily, it now seems determined to stay closed. Sadly, I am somewhere outside of myself. Have the experiences of my life, my fears and doubts, finally destroyed my ability to feel? The drums continue, but I am lost. Even now with the ominous sounds of 'Owashi'-'Mighty Eagle', beating giant wings

to incite my soul, I am not quite connecting. On the sidelines I notice the two German truck drivers watching the performance completely in awe, but where am I? And then as if in answer to my question, there it is! Not in me, but in the reflection of a stranger set before me. I watch as this huge man is transformed, visibly shaken, pacing to and fro, unable to form words yet, just his deep breathing uniting with the rhythm of what he has just witnessed. His innocent excitement brushes against my psyche and with that comes a familiar knowing that 'All is well'. Ancient magic comes crashing up against the portal of my own being demanding entrance. In those moments it is clear – Trust – the vital element to being, flew into my soul.

The day begins with a continuous flow of interfaith - meditation, chanting, poetry, and prayer, all leading to a candlelit vigil…

As the drums mark a steady masculine energy inviting stealth for the sinews, a gentle rain falls and the soft grace of ´the feminine finds it's truly powerful and nurturing voice. Across the oceans the warmongers beat their frenzied call to violence, but here within this gathering of ancient wisdom, love and spiritual power, the drums call out for peace…

Later in the evening the drums begin with ´Kaiko´- the birth of creation. This time I cannot stop my body from moving with the rhythm. Usually I have heard it several times by now in rehearsal, but as fate would have it, here I am with a room full of mostly women, hearing it again for the first time in two years. Surely I am safe? Surely they will be feeling the same magnetic resonance course through their being…

And what if they're not?

Too late, the drums…no more thinking…suddenly there is no choice…I am galloping through cosmic skies with the crescendo that happens midway. It's a force akin to a herd of galloping wild horses, and inevitably as spirit moves I find myself inexplicably riding with them.

Every cell in my body is affected...a fiery force of freedom spirals through the wheels of light in my body...on and on... spinning into timeless galaxies, as if the rhythm could last forever...as if all hopes and dreams could be accomplished...

'Never give up'... chanting silently within.
'Believe in the magic and never give up!'

And suddenly I am not alone...by the time the piece concludes women are screaming out, releasing great cries of joy and empowerment.

They got it...they got it!!!

But of course, how could they not? Temple priestesses were all skilled at drawing from the drum, rhythms that entrained the mind to ecstatic union with the Divine...

Drumming has been a necessary and respected skill amongst holy women throughout history....

November 7, 2002, UK

And now it's as if I dreamt it all...

Back here in my little cupboard of a room piled high with painted glass and diaries; books on healing, and light...

Is my life too complex, I wonder?

I'm starting to question now what must be abandoned as I approach this next portal.

I had my three-month check up last week. No big drama one way or another since **I seem to have closed the door on the fear that this disease will be my demise.**

My body feels amazingly well, although the lump is still there.

According to Dr. Ryke Geerd Hamer's theory, a tumour occurs to encapsulate the rogue cells until the immune system can return to normal, so I am not too concerned since I feel so well.

The German oncology MD Ryke Geerd Hamer had worked as a doctor of internal medicine for 15 years, five as a professor and a few in his own private practice, he had also devoted some time to the invention of specialized medical tools, when, in 1978, his 19-year-old son Dirk was shot, unexpectedly, by a madman. Naturally, the event shocked Hamer deeply. And as if this tragedy wasn't enough, around a year later, he received another unexpected message - he'd developed testicular cancer, despite having been healthy all his life. His wife later developed cancer too. Needless to say, Hamer was devastated because of all this loss, but, as we all do in a state of shock, he also started to think. Why did everything seem to come at once?

Now being a cancer doctor, Hamer had access to numerous medical resources and patient journals. While fighting his own cancer, he started reading his patients' journals and test results with new eyes. What he slowly found was something revolutionary, namely that both his own and all his patients' brain tomographies clearly showed a "focus"; a round field, exactly at the place in the brain where the nerves extended down to the organ in the body which was cancerated! What was more, when Hamer talked to his patients, he found that all of them, without exception, had experienced a sudden, deep shock some time before they developed their cancer. It turned out that the fields visible on the tomography slides had always been interpreted as either artifacts created by the equipment, or "cancer metastases" in the brain. No one had dared suggesting that perhaps the brain foci actually were the causes of the cancers, and that perhaps, in turn, the shocks all cancer patients had experienced actually were the causes of the brain foci. But Hamer did, and a clear picture started to take form: Emotional shocks were the causes of the brain foci (because all other alternatives after careful research were ruled out), and the brain foci, in turn, the causes of the cancers.

~ *And So We Heal* ~

And all sorts of different substances said to be causes of cancer turned out not to cause cancer, but indeed, to complicate it, often severely, and paradoxically, medical chemicals and equipments used for CANCER TREATMENT proved to top the list! Likewise, Hamer found that the absolutely most common shocks preceding discovery of so-called cancer metastases, were, in fact, those induced by the verdicts of various cancer diagnoses. Metastases, it turned out, were nothing else than results of new shocks, and not, as generally thought, the result of blood stream-travelling tumor cells - which also explained why no one had ever seen any such swim around there in the first place. Actually, it also explained why animals practically never get "metastases"; you see, animals don't understand diagnoses.

Of course, being a cancer doctor himself, Hamer was stunned by all this, but he couldn't deny what clearly became evident to him, and he was forced to accept that the words "psychosomatic" and "iatrogenic" comprised so much more than was previously thought.

Later, Hamer discovered that not only cancers, but also the cancer "equivalents" ulcer and hypofunction were elicited through this same pathway. He also found that Nature handles the development and recuperation of all these conditions perfectly on its own (except in rare, extreme cases), and that all that's needed is to support the individual through the stages. Practical help, psychotherapy, biologically correct nutrition and fasting, those became the cornerstones of the new treatment.

In addition, Hamer discovered why Nature responds with canceration when faced with a shock. The medical hypothesis about meaningless, malevolent and madly multiplying cells turned out to be nonsense - instead, a picture of cunning usage of a highly controlled form of cell division took form.

Hamer named his revolutionary new medicine just that, "New Medicine" (NM), because the revelation was new, even though, of course, this scheme of Nature had been there forever.

So could thus any sudden, deep shock at all start cancer? Yes, cancer or its equivalents. And not only could, it will. Here's the core of Hamer's discovery; every unexpected event that had upset his patients had caused cancer (or ulcer, or hypofunction) in them. All shocks, in all patients - not merely "most". This consistency was a refreshingly new observation within medical research; up to that point, whenever different suspected cancer triggers had been examined, merely "some" or "most" of the individuals in the test groups had presented with the disease - which had led to long lists of things established to be associated with cancer, but not really causing it, since the effect was never 100 %. The shocks discovered by Hamer, however, proved to elicit cancer or cancer equivalents 100 % of the time, so finally, the word "cause" could be used with full correctness.

Hamer named these cancer/ulcer/hypofunction triggering shocks DHS conflicts ("Dirk Hamer Syndrome" in honor of his son), and they are all, as said, unexpected experiences which upset us, although they may be of very varying intensity, some peter out in a minute, others can last for years. Now these conflicts do not belong to our intellectual realm, instead they are what Hamer called biological, because historical evolution has to be understood since the conflicts are analogous in humans and animals. We have to look past our intellectual conflicts or problems, DHSes are conflicts of a fundamentally different kind. Our bodily responses to them are, by Nature, implanted in the archaic, involuntary program of our brain. Our thoughts have no say here. In fact, the conflict has already associatively hit a fraction of a second before we even begin to think. It's automatic, and it's not negative, on the contrary, it helps us to adapt. For example, the breast gland of a female immediately cancerates when her young gets injured, helping her milk production along and thus her young heal. The kidney collecting tubes cancerate right away when the organism risks drying out - in cases of "refugee" traumas, the urine becomes highly concentrated. In a territory-loss conflict, the inner layer of the vessels supplying the heart promptly ulcerate, allowing the heart to pump more blood to the muscles in preparation for a hard fight. And so on. This mechanism is hence both automatic and AIDING, and nothing we can or should fight in any way. On the contrary, we should, by natural means, help it and support it, so that its course runs smoothly.

Actually 99.9% of the time I am jubilantly positive.

It's just that there is never enough time to complete all that I have on my list in any given day. I am beginning to wonder if I must seriously accept the fact that my glass painting days are drawing to a close.

I still want to express myself through art and looking back there have been so many phases of my artistic expression- acting, writing, painting, healing.

I guess the bottom line is that I am frustrated because I am not focusing on my priority at present: to complete this book. It takes all my time and energy to complete my regime everyday. By the time I get through the juicing and meal prep, and enemas, the day is half gone, and then it's time to start the whole cycle again.

I cast another favourite oracle, the Runes:

> ANSUZ: Hope, inspiration, words, transformation
> INGWAZ: Rest, internal growth, gestation
> DAGAZ: Awakening, awareness, hope, happiness

December 2, 2002, UK

It's my birthday, and I wake up from a dream with the words and melody of 'My Sweet Lord' on my lips and an image of George Harrison in my mind's eye. It accompanies a vague dream in which I remember going to some of his devotees to tell them that George had crossed over safely after he died.

~ And So We Heal ~

Winter draws in...but not too cold as yet...spirits remain high. So much has happened in one year and I am truly grateful for all my 'purification'. I understand it all now and can begin this new phase of my life with courage.

Javier called to say 'Felicidades'. Not too much was said really, but 'words' never the less. Words I had thought lost forever.

I am glad I stood strong to preserve our delicate friendship. As mysterious as my longing is for him, there is a treasured part of my soul that likes to think that what we have may be as profound as love gets. Certainly it has survived terrible pain.

Reflecting on memories of my life in Hollywood makes me smile now - somehow they are beginning to come full circle. I saw Lindsay Wagner, 'The Bionic Woman' in Geneva. I chatted to her briefly reminding her that not only was I her stand-in on a film, I also played the part of a nurse delivering her baby on a TV movie, 'Callie and Son'. Linda Gray of 'Dallas' was there also, and Linda Evans, who saddened me deeply when I saw what botox had done to this once extremely beautiful woman. (Sorry Linda!) God knows what might have happened to me if fame had indeed knocked on my door back then.

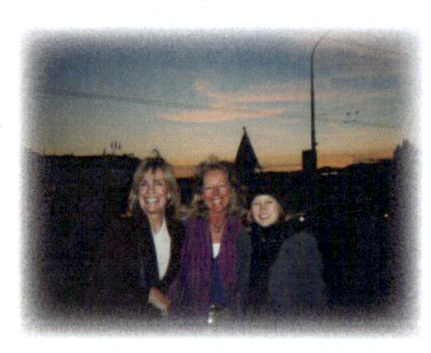

I begin to treasure the path my own life has taken.

As I appreciate these wintry days I can feel the wind whispering, that with the New Year, much change is coming...

Positive...
Transformational...
Loving...
Supportive...
Vital

~ And So We Heal ~

December 22, 2002, UK

All the '2's as it were! Winter Solstice is upon us and now we must turn to the promise of spring with its warmth.

My Christmas miracle is that I am finally off to Barcelona again January 23rd. Javier has agreed to meet again after seventeen months apart. It is a chance for us to heal this dreadful wound that was at once my pain and my salvation. I walk towards this date with trust in the almighty.

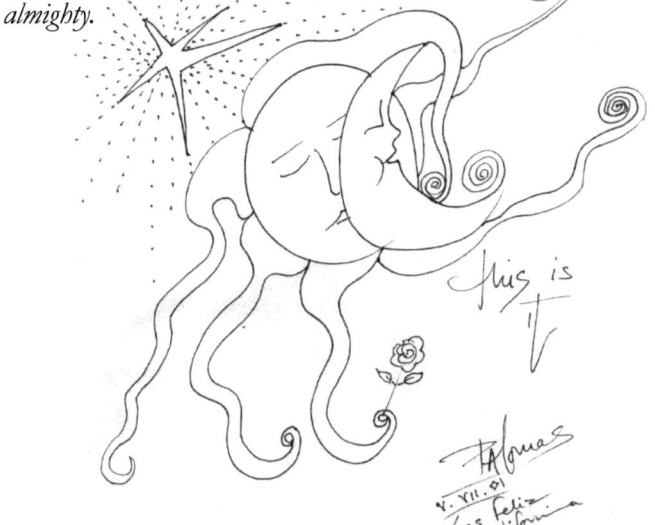

Somehow having this lump in my breast helps me to come to terms with the past, and as the healing journey continues I begin to embrace new life. I am free…and so is he, but that is just one level…there are still so many layers to this story.

I rejoice then in sharing this healing time
wherein the "crystalline" lump shall continue to dissolve
and lose ALL dominion over my well being.
I bless the lump and release it into caring hands that will destroy
it with mercy.

(Strangely, I am suddenly thinking of the character Golam in 'Lord of the Rings'. I am sure these regular injections of mistletoe are affecting my train of thought. I've really noticed a heightened awareness of nature, especially walking through the back woods behind the family home.)

January 3, 2008, UK
The New Year is here with days of sunshine and frost biting at fingers and toes. I have been healing my hands this winter. Quite a dreadful sight and painful tightness of the muscles, so much so that I thought my hands were becoming arthritic. The truth is I need to be in sunshine, to warm my flesh.

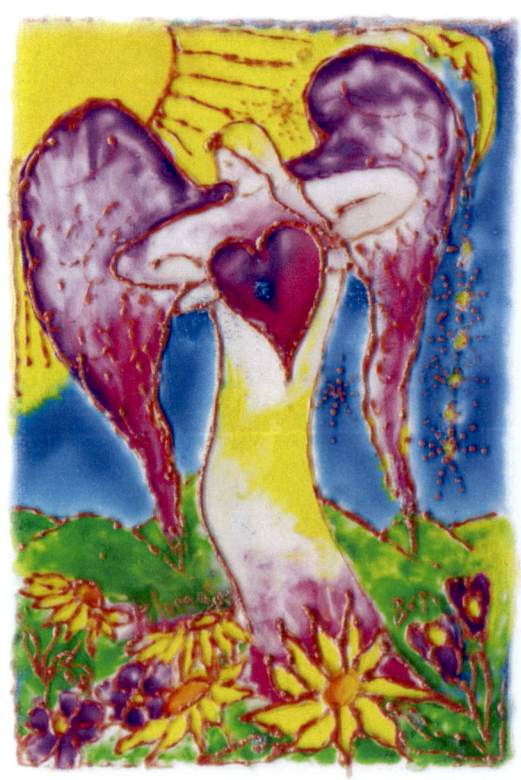

~ And So We Heal ~

January 18, 2003, UK
A few days before I leave for Barcelona I shuffle the 'Sacred Path Cards' invoking spirit to try to understand what this energy is between Javier and I.

Three times in a row I pick: **THUNDER BEINGS** - *USABLE ENERGY:*

Thunder - beings that give us the fire from the sky,
Energy for Mother Earth,
Divine creation flies through the air to touch us
Electrifying change, bringing loves true essence into our hearts again.
The Thunder Beings make up the love call of the Sky Nation. Fire sticks, or lightening bolts are a rare gift from the sky to the earth mother.
Divine Union of earth and sky. The host of lovers who give energy to Mother Earth. The fire sticks create a bridge between the two lovers and are a physical expression of their love for one another. Since our Earth Mother is magnetic in nature, she has need of the electrical energy supplied by the Thunder-beings. As the cloak of Father Sky covers the Earth Mother in a mantle of blue each day, we 'two-leggeds' see the beauty of his love for her when the cloud people form and the thoughts of their combined ideas take physical shape. 'Hail-lo-way-ain' in Seneca is the language of love. If a fire stick touches Mother Earth in one area, the electricity may travel great distances to re-energise those places that need male energy that Father Sky supplies. The Thunder beings can bring us courage to master our sense of loss by seeing the expansive plan.

Chapter Seven

Back to Barcelona

> A single beat from the heart of a lover is capable of drowning out a thousand sorrows
>
> Naquib Mahfouz

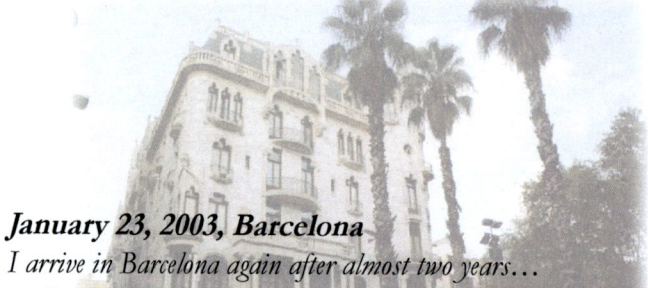

January 23, 2003, Barcelona
I arrive in Barcelona again after almost two years…
I come to heal. It is the beginning of an unknown journey and I need courage to face Javier after so much unspoken stuff has gone on between us. Somehow I had given him the wrong arrival time and he is at the airport two and a half hours early. Not an ideal start. He looks well and I immediately know that 'Yes', I will always love him, but I have come to release my heart from this never-ending yearning.

We seem to pick up where we left off, chatting over a few ciders in the local bar; but things have changed.

Last time we were together it was he that was healing from his heart operation. Now it is I, with this hard lump in my breast, threatening my life. I must use all the energy available to shrink the tumour and move forward with my life.

Javier is currently living with his mother so I have booked a room in a local pensión. Unfortunately it's on a busy street, and I toss and turn all night, drifting in and out of sleep, waking up freezing cold to fill my hot-water bottle. This area that I once loved so much, seems a little sad now, or maybe it's just that I miss the old familiar warmth of having his arms around me. But I am determined to not be emotional this trip. I must keep my calm, my strength, my positive attitude. I pray to Archangel Michael for help.

Upon waking, I do feel better and remember one of several dreams:
Javier and Shimizu, one of the lead drummers from Shumei Taiko are making circles around me. It is very prophetic and I know it.

Even though I have promised myself that I will be strong and accept all that this journey brings, in my heart of hearts, there still resides this mystery of what we two, Javier and Pauline, are to each other. I shout out to the 'sky gods' for help.

January 24, 2003, Barcelona
Moving hotels helps with the noise factor, and later I go to 'La Llibreria de Los Angeles', a local 'Angel' art and book shop, where I sell some of my art. I am confronted by a huge wall-size painting of an angel by Marta Cabeza and I become emotionally overwhelmed by it. Maria Pilar, the owner is very sweet. She hugs and kisses me, making me feel very protected, and arranges for me to attend a workshop with Marta the next day.

That night Javier and I finally lie with each other in my bed – don't ask me how we managed to end up there! We take time to massage each other gently and he puts his hand over my breast as I ask him to and

119

says a prayer. It is very sweet, and later we make love, but there is not the same depth of feeling from me.

I find myself holding back, not wanting to give too much for fear of being hurt again. Even so, it is the warmth I have been searching for and the moments when we touch each other's hands and feet under the sheets as we wrestle with sleep are perhaps for me the hidden treasure.

I want so much to help Javier open his heart to me but I am afraid he has locked it up and this time I cannot find the key...

January 26, 2003, Barcelona

I awake today after another relatively good sleep. It is eight-thirty a.m. but I manage to drift back off for another hour.
Yesterday I ate some lamb in an Argentinean restaurant with Javier. Later I wandered around on my own trying to digest; not so much the lamb, but what my life is all about. Strangely, the lamb had a good grounding effect on me, and apart from being spicier than I would have liked, was quite enjoyable.

In retrospect, I realise that all the dreams I've been having are actually now revealing their meaning to me, in subtle ways, sometimes years later.

So many times in dreams I find myself with Javier, seated around a table, seemingly talking...Now in reality as I sit here and there talking with him attempting to find answers, he is apparently very clear in how he wants his life to be, and he does not want to make any kind of commitment to a future together. I must contemplate the fact that I may be in love with a dream that can simply never ever be. Even though in my heart of hearts I know that Javier is most always in two minds about things - his birth sign is Gemini (the twins) and I know from the past that he is always changing his mind.

Tears have fallen, as I bravely face the idea of letting him go, but my equilibrium has for the most part kept its delicate balance, and I am in control. Examining the reasons why I need and want this relationship so much, they all dissolve as having no real substance. When all the dissolving and coagulating etc, is done, what remains is simply a mystery...the quintessence of feelings... the touch of another...someone to love and care about...

Human feelings...honest and simple...easy as that!

Perhaps part of the puzzle is that I once thought Javier to be slipping away, on deaths door, before his operation, and I vowed to love him always.

But now it is my own body that I must heal, and perhaps this is all part of the path that I must walk alone. Oh God, how difficult it is. I know that once I leave Spain I will have further strength, but for the moment I only have my day-to-day feelings...confusing as they sometimes are.

January 27, 2003, 'Sagrada Familia Cathedral', Barcelona

I am again filled with tears as I gaze up at the front façade with its many sculptures ascending to the heavens as it were. Strangely, I see myself in several images... parts of myself, my pain, and my story.

Walking into the interior I am attracted to the bright colours of the stained glass windows. When I try to hold back the thoughts and emotions, I hear a voice singing inside my head, "Love will come again..."

But I don't want love to come again....not a new love....what's wrong with this one!

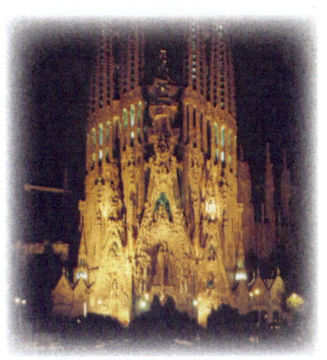

~ And So We Heal ~

Javier's image appears before me again and I am still seeking some clear answer as to what our relationship has been about all these years, if it hasn't been about everlasting love, and never giving up! On and on my mind rambles...Oh what a child I am. What a life I lead! For now, I must remember to allow these feelings to come. They help to dissolve the tumour, I am sure. It's part of the alchemical process of 'Dissolution', and I remind myself that this journey is all about healing.

Healing is feeling and feeling is dealing and dealing is healing!
...and ...well you get the picture!

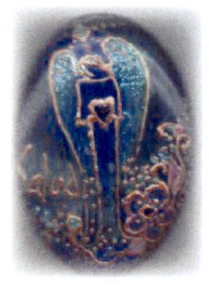

By the time I reach 'Organic', my favourite vegetarian restaurant, its four pm, and I'm quite weak and hungry. Thank God for the carrot juice and healthy food. Later I take some 'Touchstones' to 'Arunchala', a local philosophical bookshop. The angel touchstones I've started painting inspired by my visit to Montserrat last year are becoming quite popular now, but a businesswoman I am not. Inevitably I give away more than I manage to sell.

I'm still in the bath at the hotel when Javier arrives half an hour early. Trying to suppress my true feelings is not easy, and I do my best to comply with his desire that we not complicate our relationship at this time, but the truth is there is a constant dialogue going on in my head.

I will never be able to NOT love Javier; this I know, but since destiny has dealt this card to me I must try to work with it as best I can. It will only cause more harm if I explode into a mad rage, and threaten never to see him again.

**Sadness gives way to joy!
A familiar pattern in my life
I am unafraid and face life with such excitement!**

~ *And So We Heal* ~

> When we truly come to terms with sorrow, a great and unshakeable joy is born in our hearts
>
> Allegra Taylor

January 28, 2003, The way to Montserrat

I awake knowing full well that I ate too many dates last night. The sugar has left me with swollen eyes. Luckily I have the coffee enema, and soon after I am starting to feel better, even though I still have this sad feeling knowing that my journey to Spain will soon be over.

I allow more tears to fall and once more invoke the assistance of Archangel Michael.

Today I am going to Montserrat. The last time was around Easter in April of 2001. It was a very moving experience then. I remember standing in line with hundreds of others to see the statue of the 'Black Madonna and Child'

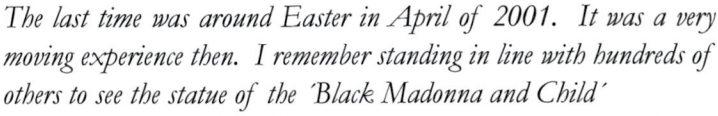

Arriving around midday, it is even more impressive than I remember. I have to put on sunglasses because tears are beginning to fall again. The sun is still quite strong above the mountain peaks, but it is cold in the shade as I make my way to the Hotel Abat Cisnero, where I have booked a room. Room thirty-three on the third floor brings an unexpected smile to my face. It's enormous and beautifully kept, with a view over the plaza to the monastery. Down below I can see my

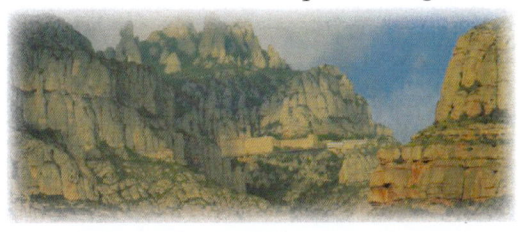

~ And So We Heal ~

favourite portals, and as soon as I drop my bags I'm off out, but not before noticing the painting over the desk. In it a woman stands ready to take a bath. She has uncovered her right breast. It's beautiful and I take this as a good omen, and scurry off to see the Madonna and child.

Stepping into the monastery, bells start to chime and I realise that I am completely alone; so different from the last time I was here at Easter with the throngs of people. I'm able to appreciate the magnificent sculptures now and am deeply affected. It's all so surreal, this great exhilaration I feel…like a welcoming back from beyond the veils. It feels as if I am in an old movie where the heroine has returned to the monastery after being in the outside world. In fact, it is the very movie that has haunted me through much of my life, "The Miracle". My mother took me to see it when I was a young girl, and it left an indelible impression on me. Carol Baker played the nun, I remember, who left the order to follow her heart, with Roger Moore, the young soldier, whom she had fallen in love with. He died, and she went on to love again, a bullfighter amongst others. Each one dropping by the wayside until she returned to the monastic life where it was revealed that the statue of the Virgin Mary had come alive to take her place in the convent whilst she was away in the outside world. I have searched in vain to find a copy of this film to see if it still impacts me in the same way. I used to think of it a lot when I lived a semi-monastic life in Japan.

Here I was again with the nun thing!

Now as I find myself flying through the chapel I am charged with a great light, realizing that there is no one else in sight. I can indulge my emotions as the damn tears begin to spring forth. The beautiful alabaster stairway of angels, all shapes and sizes, takes my breath away, and the colourful mosaics appear like jewels as I wind my way up the narrow stairs to find the black Madonna and Child. Since there is still no one in sight, I allow the tears to flow freely and with them my prayer.

~ And So We Heal ~

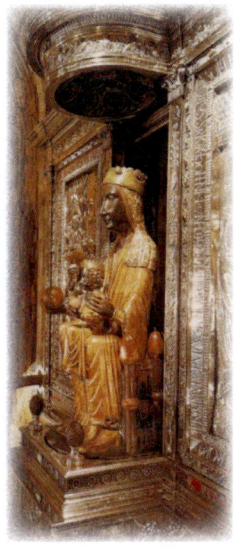

'Dear God, I need so much healing', I am unabashed in my imploring.

My hand reaches out to the sphere that the Madonna is extending. I softly touch it and then make my way to the room behind wherein magnificent stained-glass windows illuminate everything. A powerful statue of St George with sword uplifted, invokes a silent scream that forces itself through my mouth, whilst all the while the tears are falling from my eyes. Allowing this great release cleanses my heavy heart, and later as I sit and gaze upward at the eight golden angels that are encircling me, I realise why I needed to come here again; to be immersed in this healing energy.

**It is time for the tumour to leave my body.
I am beseeching the gods now.**

January 29, 2003, Montserrat

Last night I walked amongst the stars breathing in the clear blue air. Once again I feel that I am alone here. It invokes feelings of the sacred mountain 'Misono' where I lived in Japan. Attending the seven o'clock service in the chapel and listening to the famous boys' choir, yet more torrents of tears came to cleanse my soul. I sleep like a baby following a late supper.

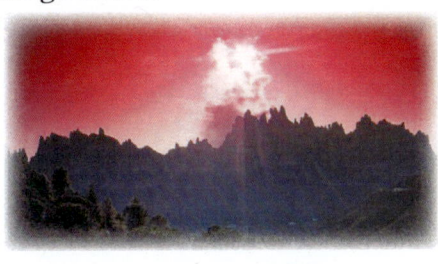

The sound of bells herald the early morning as I open the curtains, to find a new moon hanging in a familiar silver crescent, with a bright star above it.

I slept an hour or so more, just because I could, and remember a dream:

~ And So We Heal ~

Every time a bell rang I went to get a drink of water. It was Alan Imai, an old Japanese friend, himself a minister, who was serving me.

The golden sun has risen high above the distant lavender-blue mountains, flooding my room with warmth and healing. Now with this bright new day I know that I can move forward with my life and my health. I prepare my morning enema, and with it a chance to reflect and meditate on the grace of this whole journey. Afterwards a breakfast of orange juice, green barley drink, oatmeal, flax and soy, and I feel well fortified; however there is still room for the hotel's breakfast of forbidden delights. Cheese... buttered rolls... coffee! It seems that all those tears have given me an enormous appetite.

Returning to my room, I sit with naked breasts exposed to the sun, and contemplate the day's agenda. Something has 'spiritized' inside me. The 'all knowingness', I came in search of - a familiar homecoming to my higher self

There is a lot of construction going on this week; cranes swing back and forth, hammers pound and the sounds of men's voices echo through the mountains, but none of it bothers me. In fact it is all quite nurturing. I don't seem to need the silence as I once did; part of me recognizes that my work belongs in the outside world. No more nuns' roles for me!

Caressing my breasts, I feel that they are both fine. When I used a pendulum the other day to ask if my disease was in regression the answer was 'yes'. I do believe it to be so and have done so for many months now.

Once again it is this aspect that I seek to share with others, **this all-knowing / know thyself realisation that needs to be nurtured.**

What I feel now running through the cells of my body as I simply caress my own self, is a reminder to me of the

~ And So We Heal ~

Divine presence within us all.
I feel that I can reach out and extend my energy to others now, and more than ever I ask for the strength, grace and wisdom to follow through with completing this book.

Part of me wishes to stay here a little while longer, but there is a bigger part of me that wants to see Javier and share the revelations of what I have just experienced.

This is always what my heart desires, to share my experiences with those beloved to me.

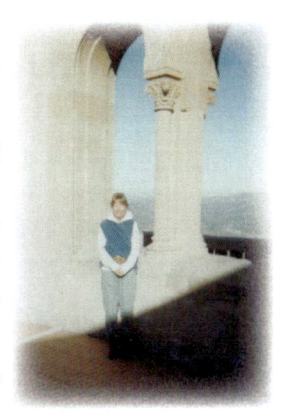

I truly feel that I have found the gold again.

To the ancient alchemist, everything in the universe is part of the Divine art of making gold...Ultimately, the 'great work', as alchemy was known, transformed true seekers to a new level of being.

IMAGINATIO or the act of imagining was a physical activity that could be channelled into the cycle of material changes. The alchemist related himself not only to the unconscious but also directly to the very substance that he hoped to transform through the power of imagination. It is a concentrated extract of life forces. Through the seven stages of alchemical transformation we arrive at coagulation - The 'Ultima materia' of the Soul.

Imagine the wellness

Below me in the plaza, tourists and pilgrims are gathering. They have been coming here since 880 ad, when according to legend, the image of the mother of God was found in a cave in the mountain. As the ever-present sound of bells ring out I allow myself to indulge in the absolute awe of what the faith of people has created here.

~ *And So We Heal* ~

Returning to the outside world I find that President Bush has just declared war on Iraq!

I did return back to Barcelona that day and Javier and I spent more time together before I left for England. We had taken the first step in mending what had been broken.
Back in the UK, I would try now to forge ahead with my life without having too many expectations…

February 5, 2003, UK
I am back in Birkenhead riding on top of a double-decker bus on my way to reflexology in Liverpool with Pam Shepherd, at the Linda McCartney Clinic.

It is exactly one week ago that I was awakened to the bright healing light of sunrise at Montserrat, and after my time with Javier, I feel that I have grounded 'the beloved'. 'She' no longer feels the need to be held in the warmth of the lover…for she is the lover.

Looking back at my writings over the last three years since re-uniting with Javier, I can now recognize more easily the person I am. My life, my purpose. Having set for myself the task of telling my story, I shall have faith that I can accomplish it, and as always invoke the assistance of Divine guidance to support this work.

As I begin to prepare to take a trip to America, to spend some time at the Optimum Health Institute in San Diego, my mind finds me caught between worlds once more. The past and the future melt into one and I am whole again feeling free and filled with the light and love of truth, as I continue on this path that opens up like a jewelled portal…
The sun is shining, golden and warm,
the skies blue with puffy clouds change from moment to moment.
Soft flurries of snow leave the streets shining silver
and the trees sparkle with jewels.

~ *And So We Heal* ~

I am full of bliss today.
Here in the present a new courage stiffens my sinews
and with the help of many

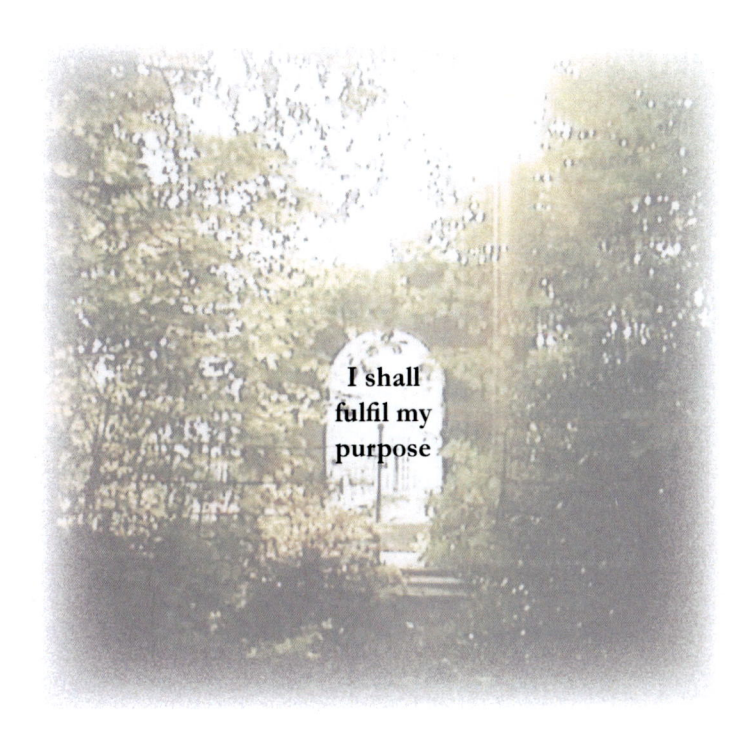

**I shall
fulfil my
purpose**

Chapter Eight

Advance

> Take your medicine bundle and all of the strengths it represents and charge forward. The advance can be on any level. Your spiritual physical mental and emotional healings are understood through life's experiences. You can now approach your destiny with every feather you have earned marking your past victories and see the destiny you have chosen emerging before you.
>
> Sacred Path Medicine cards

February 5, 2003, UK

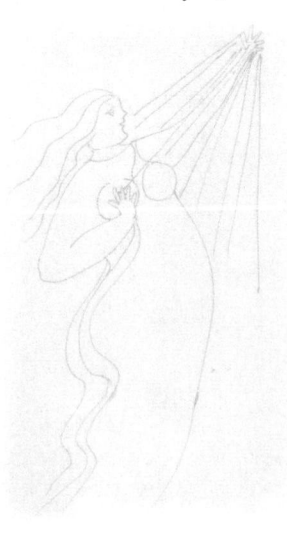

I went for my 'lymphatic drainage' treatment with Helen. Bless her for all the hard work over the last year, helping me to detoxify and re-energise my lymph system. I stared down at my legs, and could actually love them for once. God knows, I have spent a lifetime with bad circulation. Finally I feel like I can have the body I always wanted. Of course I have to accept the fact that I am older now, and a fifty-one year old woman at that. Did I say 51? Suddenly just writing this down, a door opens and I am now ready to accept this! Life is too short to think of the past.

~ *And So We Heal* ~

I put my right hand on my right breast and feel the hard lump within… It does not threaten me anymore. All fear subsides within the safe all-knowing of my indomitable faith. I pick up my banner and move forward.

I AM WELL
I AM THAT
I AM

February 12, 2003, UK

My dream the night before brought flowing blood and then my period came the next morning, the soft red earthy coloured redness reminding me that I am alive.

I must put my energy into the birth of this book. It seems to sprout new shoots in my being. This 'being' that is the vessel of who I am. This instrument desires to nurture feelings that demand to be released into the world through words.

February 14, 2003, UK

I receive a Valentine e-mail message from Javier! A beautiful drawing of a human heart pumping away. Searching for words amongst thousands I find these to send to him:

"Lighting a light to carry me on, the ancients call softly, 'remember the song'. Be of the earth, of the moon and the stars. Be in your heart wherever you are.

Be in your heart wherever you are."

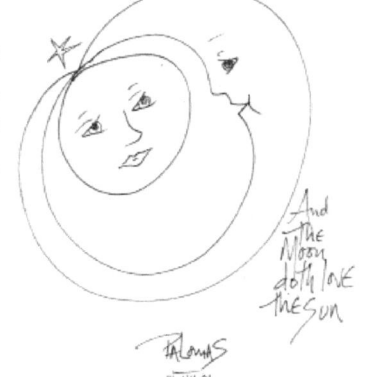

~ And So We Heal ~

As today is St. Valentines day the portal to my true heart opens up and I allow myself to speak of love and kisses…of warmth and touch. I allow myself to remember hands touching underneath sheets. One night of pleasure, that seems so unreal now.

Was it all a dream? Did we share laughter and tears, as always?
Yes it is true…we found the magic portal and shared our lives a little.
And yes, things have changed. For the better I feel.
Honesty does that…
Let us always be honest.
Let us always be friends.

February 18, 2003, UK

I went for reflexology yesterday with Pam Shepherd at the Linda Mc Cartney clinic. This ancient art of foot massage works with the body's meridian lines and Pam's dedication to helping her patients is a real blessing at the hospital.

In 1989 confronted with terrible pain following a back injury Pam went in search of alternative ways to relieve her pain, since the medication available at the time was not adequate. She took several therapeutic courses and eventually was able to use what she had learnt in the intensive care unit to help calm patients who became agitated with surgical procedures. She slowly disseminated her knowledge to other nurses and word spread leading Pam to become a palliative care specialist, resulting in the Royal Liverpool Hospital becoming one of the first in the country to recognize the importance of such care for patients.

As always her gentle touch evokes the bright colours of the chakras, which swirl through my consciousness bringing balance and healing. Later after the session she tells me that she saw lots and lots of feathers around me, and asked if they were of any significance.

~ And So We Heal ~

'But of course'- I recount the many times feathers appear to me and how their symbolism is a sign of hope to me.

It has become very frosty of late, but I am very energised after the session and treat myself to long awaited fish and chips. It feels good to have a nice hot meal out instead of my own little cold packed lunch of 'same old, same old healthy fare'.

I take a bus into Aigburth, in Liverpool to visit my friend Jane Lawn who has just returned from the Czech Republic where she's been undergoing tests for an alternative approach to treating her breast tumour. It seems the findings have revealed hidden virus and weakened immune system, and she is embarking on another regime - very expensive but designed to regulate her system. She has tried lots of different approaches, and I always support her choices and determination. I cannot even begin using this protocol, as it is too expensive.

Jane and I have a lot in common; both around the same age, diagnosed the same year. Both of us artists, Jane is an American living in England, and I English, having lived in America. We make a good team, always investigating the latest natural approaches to our 'condition'. It helps so much to have a kindred spirit to share the experience. She insists that I try out her ozone machine and I wish that I could have one for myself, but again, it's not just the expense, $2000 or so, but the space to keep all this equipment.

I have been feeling new sensations in my chest area and try to remain positive, but last night before I go to bed I find two little lumps around my neck area. I hope it's not much to worry about, but of course one does. I slept well however, and this morning
I decide to push on through courageously...

March 3, 2003, UK

Once again I have a flare-up with the hands. It's a bit of an ongoing dilemma actually. Of course immersing my hands in cold water all the time washing my veggies doesn't help, but I soldier on... At least this time the skin has not been punctured so I just try to keep the circulation going with massage. I've increased the carrot apple and ginger juice because of the little lump I've discovered in my neck.

March 4, 2003, UK

I have to accept that the book has its own schedule and I can't stress myself thinking that I have to rush it; especially now that I am preparing to go to California in two weeks.

My treatments and supplements are so expensive and I trust that all shall be provided for. It's more important that I continue to heal.

As I mentioned at the beginning, I had very little money, and yet despite that, I can honestly say that I felt that I had everything I needed.

Most importantly I had the love of my family and friends and I was able to appreciate the miraculous power of nature...

Each day brings simple pleasures- the spring flowers poking through- daffodils, crocus and little bunches of snowdrops unexpected on the path delight my eye. Gracie our little dog is a good old buddy, a soft, white, fluffy bundle to snuggle into and baby.

March 6, 2003, UK

When I feel my breast to assess the lump, it mostly feels the same except during the weeks leading to my period when my breasts are heavier and so give the impression of more fluid around it. The node under my right arm stays the same and although it is quite annoying to feel the new nodes on my neck I try to pay more attention to keeping the lymph flowing in that area. Dry skin brushing helps and Jane is encouraging me to delve into Urine therapy- there are so many accounts of its healing properties in almost all cultures. It's actually quite amazing!

I've stopped worrying about the lump in the neck. Surely all this detoxification must naturally clog up the nodes from time to time, since it is their job to carry toxins in and out of the body, and so if I keep

~ And So We Heal ~

up the regime my enhanced immune system will keep any intruding cells from setting up camp.

I simply must hold good thoughts

I light a candle for Nelda Brown - 3.3.2003…another dear friend has lost her valiant battle.

March 24, 2003, California
This morning I could feel strong purple light during my meditation. I am also bringing in the silver sword again to pierce the lump. I must make more of a conscious effort now with my visualisations.

As the spring pushes forth so, too, my own determination and courage …

I am at the 'Optimum Health Institute' near San Diego California – Arrived from England last Monday. One week has passed, despite the horrible reality of the war in Iraq. I am on a retreat here to clear my soul and shrink the tumour. Not sure what comes first at this point although I am adjusting to the regime and finding humour in everything. Its wheat grass, wheat grass, and more wheat grass…I sleep well.

March 26, 2003, California
It is both rejuvenating, but draining three days of juice fasting. Still I'm not complaining, as all in all it is a challenge and a great opportunity to detoxify, although the lump does not seem to have changed. I'm doing wheat grass enemas also, and colonic irrigation. I've had several wheat grass poultices on the breast also to draw out the toxins but my skin has been quite itchy, with a rash all

In my meditations I still find Javier and my daydreams create a life in Spain.

~ And So We Heal ~

over my body, even my face. Despite feeling like 'the hulk' I am meeting very nice people and there is a great natural attitude to healing. We are all in the same boat so one green hulk supports the other!
I cheated today and had a very small handful of sunflower seeds… Am so looking forward to solid food!

And all will be well,
And all manner of things will be well.
Julian of Norwich

May 8, 2003, UK
My homeopath Dr Richardson reminds me that today is 'Julian of Norwich' day. He has described my own essence as resembling that of this woman mystic of her time. Here we go with the nun theme again!
These days are still spent with detoxification most of the time, although I do allow myself the time to feel like a normal person when I go into the city… that is, I allow myself to indulge in a few cravings, a cheese and onion pasty, a bag of chips, or a de-café soy latte here or there. Nothing too outrageous! After all this time being so good, I have to have these days where I can just say- F---it! I'm going to enjoy myself. Otherwise life becomes all about living just to fetch the next bag of carrots, and boil up the next pan of coffee.

When I leave Dr. Richardson's office a small 'touchstone' falls out of my pocket – LOVE LIFE, it says… and so I rejoice!!

I do proclaim today that I shall continue on with this quest to heal.

~ And So We Heal ~

May 17, 2003, UK
I was beginning to think that putting pen to paper would elude me forever...

These days have been days wherein my body is free to heal with no pressing 'schedule' or doctors appointments.

There was a profound sense of 'healing' today, and I was able to envision glimpses of my breasts appearing very healthy and youthful. Taking time to examine the tumour... its shape and size have remained the same for the last six months. The edges, the general shape is so familiar to me now, mostly as an egg shape.

I choose to see it as an egg that is little by little crystallizing and leaving my body.

Sometimes I imagine I can hear the 'clink' sound of it like a thin bullet being dropped into a vessel. Sometimes I look at the possibility of an extraction, a necrotic- dying of the tumour – slipping out of me.

How exactly would the 'tumour' exit the body I wonder?
I was to find out, but just not now.

May 21, 2003, UK
This English weather is not warming to the bones but I breathe in vital green energy from the surrounding green land.

Sunshine and clouds, showers upon us...
Somehow knowing there are blue skies above...
simply knowing- is enough to remember the mountain of faith.

I spread the RUNES:

Gestation
Rest – internal growth
Contained, isolated separation, which is absolutely necessary to any transformational process. Here in solitude & stasis new growth arises.

~ And So We Heal ~

Deep level gestation of new power. Rest, let things gestate to be brought forth at the right time in full maturity.
PATIENCE…Listen to yourself.
A time of stasis to be followed by Fertile Dynamism …a potential state awaiting…ACTIVATION.

May 28, 2003, UK

Rejoice --- the pen desires to move across the page!
So many thoughts fill my mind when I curl up on the bedroom floor, buttocks naked to the summer breeze dancing through my familiar bedroom window. The neighbourhood noises, lovely and friendly…voices of children, so many blonde haired young ones these days, five to a family sometimes…

When I saw my oncologist Alison Waghorn last Friday she measured the lump and found it to be bigger, five point something. I wasn't too worried, because in truth – my truth - I don't feel it to have grown for the most part. I choose to see the glass half full of life, as opposed to half empty, you see.

I treasure these times that remind me to be grateful, to move forward, casting off other's fears that my condition is worsening.

The truth is, my journey of transformation continues, with or without the lump. In a way, the tumour serves to remind me to be gentle and calm with myself.

May 29, 2003, UK

I saw my GP, Dr Richmond this morning. He has been very supportive of my choices and taught me how to inject the mistletoe. I asked him for another referral for Osteopathy and one for acupuncture since they are fully booked at the 'Wirral Holistic'. He gave me a very forceful argument, basically saying that it was the 'Wirral Holistic Clinic' that should provide that service, and the only acupuncturist he knew had a long waiting list, and why should I be given an appointment when he normally reserved those referrals to people with chronic pain.

Oh-oh! I suddenly became very emotional and tears sprang into my eyes. Then with my blood boiling I lashed out and laid it all on the line...

"Not all pain can be measured as chronic!
There is a deep well of emotional pain inside me."

The truth is **I have been doing everything I can to heal myself***, really not costing 'the system' much at all.*

If I had gone the traditional route with chemotherapy, radiation and years of Herceptin, or some other drug that cost a fortune, I would have racked up a bill of many many many thousands by now. Surely I ranked alongside the 'chronic'. At least I wasn't asking him for a bottle of pills to mask the pain! Acupuncture is widely acclaimed nowadays. Why isn't it more readily available to those of us seeking holistic healing?

Later, I recognized that I am premenstrual and my emotions these past few days have certainly been expressing that. This is detoxification! In retrospect, I am really grateful for all my experiences and value this day. In truth, I give thanks to all my doctors, and especially appreciate Dr. Richmond's ability to see my point of view.

The NHS system is overloaded, I know this. I also know that I must take a stand for what I believe in.

I am determined to get well and hopefully be some help in improving things.

June 3, 2003, UK

Things have not been easy just now. I feel the toxins moving through my body as my cells seek to dispel all that is no longer useful to my purpose. I am filled with emotion and cry very easily, my hormones perhaps. I struggle to remain positive and understand that this is more purification. Physically there are more lumps and bumps and emotionally I think of Javier a lot.

Last night Javier's face came in a dream smiling to cheer me up. A few nights ago another dream: Javier and I were running. He was afraid and caught my arm whilst we continued hurtling forward until the terrain changed texture beneath our feet.

I long to get onto the next level with my life but am not sure what that is and where it will lead...

I trust in the Almighty to guide me and protect this path and give me courage.

Another Rune reading reveals:

YEW - Enlightenment
ENDURES BEYOND ALL THINGS
Yew is evergreen in winter.
Life in the midst of death – used to build fires, becoming the sun within.
The inner flame must be ignited then realization of inner strength will protect you from outside dangers – bring together light & dark.

Endures beyond all things!

I'll take some of that thank you!!!!

June 29, 2003, UK

I somehow found the courage to travel again and left for Paris last Thursday for the annual gathering of Shumei-jyorei practicioners in

~ *And So We Heal* ~

Europe. I always used to love travelling but since my diagnosis it now takes a giant leap of faith. I've heard it described as a shrinking of the comfort zone, which I think, hits the nail on the head. But I've found that if one can at least attempt to step outside this zone then divine providence is usually there waiting in the wings as was the case this time.

What an amazing journey. To be with my friends from Shumei, and feel their sincerity and commitment to helping the world, brought a great light into my life and infused me with a renewed vigour. Physically I did very well although it was extremely hot. My legs were quite swollen and I had a headache a lot of the time - but I knew that it was probably because of the excitement. I was just so very happy to be in Paris that I needed to indulge a little.

Thank God for the coffee enemas – I really can't say that enough!

Whilst resting on the afternoon after the meeting, I felt a beautiful green light pervade my consciousness, slowly spiralling in on me. It was a magical awakening leaving me refreshed and powerful, somehow knowing that healing was imminent.

Before leaving France I travelled to Chartres Cathedral for the spring equinox and experienced a mystical light from the sun shining through a small portal in the wall.

Walking the famous labyrinth I felt grateful to be alive and in touch with spirit.

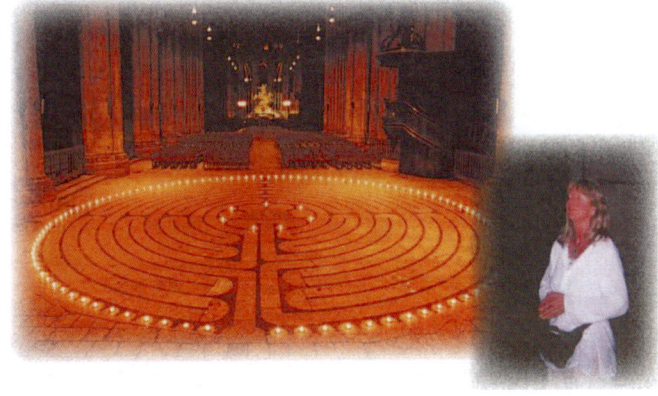

Chapter Nine
The Calling to Greece

Exciting energy is leading me to the 'Oracle', at Delphi.

I have felt Tom my old partner's presence today... tinkling bells ... awakening memory. I had so desperately wanted to take him to Greece, somehow feeling that if I could get him there in the hot sun and energy of some former life I could help him in this one.

I will fly to Crete July 22nd, spend a week there and get the ferry to Athens to make my way to Delphi. I'm planning to be there August first for the seventh anniversary of Tom's death. There are many ancient connections with the goddess energy in particular that have their roots in Crete – the Minoan civilization.

July 23, 2003, Crete

I arrived in Greece yesterday, the island of Crete, and the village of Malame to be exact. The first villager named Maleme from the Greek phrase 'Malama'-a synonym of 'gold', and shows the fertility of land and sea.

It's all quite magical really. Another healing journey, this I know without a doubt.

I slept maybe two hours and the taxi picked me up at 4.40am for a 7.40am flight from Manchester, arriving in Chania, Crete three and a half hours later.

As always I was a little nervous about the journey, especially this time because not only was I setting off alone, but I was going somewhere

~ *And So We Heal* ~

I'd never been before and not meeting anyone familiar upon arrival. All my travel over the years has been for a specific purpose – not for vacation. This time I'm on holiday – I intend to bask in the sunshine and swim in warm healing waters.

The last time I set off like this to parts unknown was about twenty months ago to Andalucia, two weeks after I was diagnosed. Still in shock and crying buckets as I remember, releasing all the pain and repressed sadness at being abandoned by Javier. This time I feel so much lighter, so much more in control of my life, so much freer.

Of all the places I could have gone in Greece it is to Crete that providence guided me. I'd booked one of those package flights and hotel deals at the last minute, and before I could 'chicken out' I was whisked into the skies and dropped into a coach from Chania airport. Any initial euphoria had by this point evaporated into feeling somewhat forlorn noticing that everybody on board had a travelling companion or companions with whom to share their expectant wonder at the start of this new Minoan adventure.

Tears began to trickle down my face as the shy little 'woe is me', voice pushed its way to the front of my consciousness, flooding into the hot flushed cheeks; familiar by-product of an inner embarrassment.

"Everybody else on board is travelling with a loved one – but I'm alone!" went the pitiful dialogue inside my head, until up from the seat in front popped a lovely smiling face asking me to help decipher her 'welcome packet' – she couldn't quite make out her destination. In the seat next to her I could barely make out the chubby white limbs and baseball cap of a child. A' he' or a 'she', it didn't matter, they had each other... I had only me. But as fate would have it we were bound for the same place, The Ledra Maleme apartments. Suddenly things were looking up as these complete strangers had unknowingly reached out and penetrated my pool of grief. On disembarking it was not long before I realized that the child was indeed female; a little unsteady on her feet as was I at this point, a pounding headache having set in. We stuck close together then, chit-chatting away as we dragged our suitcases down the long dusty country lane that housed our holiday homes.

If truth be known, I think we were all glad of friendly banter, and before we reached the reception, the woman who I assumed was the little one's mother told me that the child had just finished radiation therapy for a brain tumour. My heart skipped a beat and I was able then to share the fact that, I too had a tumour, as a way of saying that we were all on this 'magical mystery tour' together.

Suddenly I was not alone anymore; the angels had provided me with friends. And so it was that Christine, who as it turns out was the grandmother and Kirstie, the little treasure, materialized in my life with perfect timing...

There were no tears of pity for me last night, only tears of joy, as I realized that there is usually some risk involved whenever we set out to embrace changes in life.

Fear often stops us moving forward...but when we do step beyond the realms of our comfort zone. Divine Providence most surely awaits.

July 24, 2003, Crete

I awoke feeling in excellent spirits. The morning sun shines on to my balcony and I can see the turquoise Aegean Sea over the green fields and bamboo groves. My heart is filled with such gratitude for this journey. Slowly I prepare the morning coffee enema that has become such a welcome part of my routine. I decided not to bring the juicer and forgo the usual two carrot and apple juice drinks. Instead I have plenty of the green barley powder super drink and intend to have at least four a day.

Since fruit is in abundance I choose the huge black grapes, munching on the grape seeds, which have great medicinal properties. At some point I plan to do an all grape fast for a day or two, but it will not be today.

Being able to lie naked on my balcony is a welcome surprise. Fortunately it turns out to be the perfect location. The warmth of the

~ And So We Heal ~

hot Mediterranean sun penetrates deeply into my breasts. Later in the afternoon I join Kirstie and Christine on a trek to the beach. It's quite pebbly and the waves are too high to swim but we enjoy a refreshing wade and find a shady enough spot to enjoy.

Later I'm a bit annoyed to discover that the sun has burnt me, despite all efforts to keep protected. Still, it's such a temptation to feel the healing rays. Late evening I watch the sun set around eight thirty, and find myself on a bus to Platanos, the next resort, along the coast. It's full of tavernas, tourist shops and throngs of brown bodies. I surprise myself and order lamb kebabs, fried potatoes and Greek bread with a delicious red wine, and then head back to Malame at ten thirty.

My moon time has arrived so I am to take it a little easy. A night cap of Retsina and finishing off the chocolate seems well deserved, although I know that cancer cells relish such sweetness, but its not a daily habit, so rather than worry about that and the excessive salt in my dinner I decide to be grateful for it and sleep comes easily save for the odd buzz from my friend the mosquito.

I awake around seven a.m., but drift in and out of sleep until nine. The coffee enema, as always brings balance and the green drink tops up my energy, followed by delicious soaked seeds, almonds, oats, yoghurt and flaxseeds.

I decide not to sunbathe today but try to catch up with writing and maybe hop on a bus to the west, see where the day takes me. I feel great.

Meeting Kirstie and Christine at the pool I find they feel great too. Kirstie is swimming a lot and determined to recover fully from her recent operation on the tumour. On top of everything her left side had become paralysed, and she starts hormone treatment next week for her growth. What an amazing child of twelve.

She certainly inspires my own determination to be well.

~ And So We Heal ~

July 26, 2003, Crete

I have been bleeding quite heavily since yesterday. My period arrived a week early but my energy level is high.

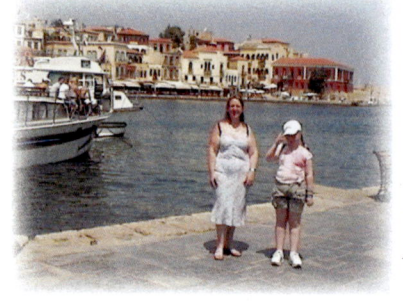

Yesterday I went with Kirstie and Christine into Chania. The heat was stifling, not a good time to be wandering around the shops but it was good to see the old town, having read so much about the history of Crete. We caught the five pm. bus up to Stavros at the head of the Akrotiri peninsular, where parts of 'Zorba the Greek' were filmed. It was so refreshing to go for a swim in the shallow bay there and watch the sun slowly set.

Riding back on the local rickety bus, the evening light was magical and a soft breeze welcoming embrace to my spirit. Kirstie kept up the pace all day and her lovely round face and happy giggles brought memories of my very first doll, Jennifer.

The electricity was off in the village when we returned after ten pm. I scrambled about by candle light trying to fix the delicious meal I had promised myself. Finishing off the red wine my head hit the pillow after midnight but it's not easy to get to sleep because of the heat. Even so, I am enjoying the heat as a chance to feel free about my body. I've had no worries about my health. All in all I keep expecting to reach down to my right breast one day and find the hard rock has disappeared.

I feel so alive, and passionate about the future.

~ And So We Heal ~

My soul feels its full potential here, and I know that I want to live in the Mediterranean climate

I still think of Javier. He is, as always, never far from my thoughts, but I realize that this could all be a happy fantasy for me. I often sense his energy as he was as a young man. Perhaps this is a way of keeping my spirit young, daydreaming like this. I don't know.

> **I don't know too much these days except that I must inspire others.**

July 27, 2003, Crete

Couldn't sleep too well last night although I went to bed early enough. I spent the afternoon at the beach and tried not to exert myself too much. The blood continues to flow and I choose to think that the tumour is breaking down and my body will exorcise it through the various fluids.

I noticed that some of my fruit has been nibbled at this morning - I must have a midnight visitor. I hope it's the four-legged variety and not the two legged, although I do find myself drawn to Mediterranean men. Coming down to the beach, knee deep in the grasses I began feeling a little low, my eyes filling easily with tears. Here I was, goats on either side of me, blue skies above and an endless turquoise sea calling to me, so why the tears?

'Snap out of it!' I tell myself.

'Be grateful for this time in Paradise.'

The truth is, there is more to release. As long as I carry this hard rock in my breast I am not free. A shadow remains across my path. My journey here is to help me unravel it...each little inch of pain... bit by bit, until I can caress my breasts, feel their healthy softness and know that I am whole again.

Standing on the pebbly shore I let the powerful waves crash up against me, refreshing water clean and cool on my body. A warm trickle of blood makes it's way between my legs and I sit in the waters letting the redness mingle with the foamy green. The tears push through again, and this time I will not stop them as it comes to torment me yet again - this sadness, and the regret at never giving birth.

Silent cries force themselves out of my mouth. Safe in the knowing that there is no one around to notice, I give in, secure in the knowledge that this too shall pass - that I shall find peace through the release. I have been within this pain before and it was a thousand times more painful. This is simply residue.

I shall survive!

The surprise however is whispered subtly - Maleme - It is here that the Germans came. Much blood was spilt on these shores.

I am reminded of the Shumei Taiko drum piece, 'Miyake', about the waves crashing against the shore - how the spirits of our ancestor's dreams exist forever, calling to us through the mysterious unknown. I acknowledge that there is a portal within my soul that allows me communion with these realms. It happened in Berlin, when the drummers were performing near the Brandenburg Gate. Perhaps it is the rhythm of this realm now that pries open my heart.

I have always been grateful to have empathy and feel the pain of others suffering, but I think the time has come now to stand strong against any further defeat to my purpose.

Documenting these words in my journal today I glance up at this very moment to a flag fluttering in the breeze - *APOLLO* is here.

July 28, 2003, Crete

I am awake this morning to the cock crowing and the sun arriving round and red on the horizon. Feeling a little rough. The wine we had at dinner last night, no doubt, and the extra salt and oil in my diet. Still, I am grateful for everything that comes my way even the midnight visitor that woke me up in the early hours. At first I thought it was trying to nibble through the paper I'd stuffed the suspect hole with, then I traced the sound around to the balcony door and spied a long tail. A lizard I thought. No such luck! My little friend was indeed a rat from the surrounding nature. There's no sense in being afraid so I shooed it off, locked the door tightly and resumed sleep, grateful to be free of mosquitoes at least.

I dreamt many, many things but cannot really remember much detail. This morning the cloud has drawn in yet again.

I've been thinking of my friend Jane Lawn since Friday knowing she was going for a consultation with the oncologist. Finally, this morning I make the phone call. I am so sad for Jane; she has been my sister in battle over this last eighteen months. We found each other through mutual necessity. Both of us have opted against surgery to heal our breast lumps through natural means. Jane has been actually doing far more than I in terms of regimes. Ozone and wheat grass among other things. A few weeks ago, due to some changes in her test results she decided to remove the lump by surgery. This morning my heart was heavy for her as she told me there was only one option, mastectomy. I try hard to offer strong positive support but there are no words left, and I know it. This has been part of my own heaviness of spirit of late. Jane is like my twin soul upon this path of healing. We each are individuals and have different history but our determination to heal our afflictions naturally has been the bond that strengthened our mutual journey.

When I hung up the phone an eerie silence stayed with me as I questioned my own future. No matter how much I believed in the choices I have made, still comes the darkness, still comes the doubt.

It is not until I sit and write of all that I am carrying inside, can I surface once more to the light.

~ And So We Heal ~

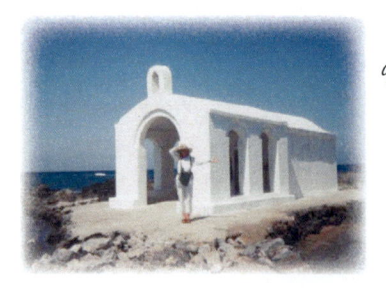

I choose one of my 'touchstones' and affirm:

Hold fast upon this Touchstone
Believe without a doubt
Herein dwells love
And miracles shall surely come about

And so it is that I welcome Joy back to my soul and courage to Journey on.

July 29, 2003, Crete

Feeling so much better today. The waves have finally been tamed and the sea is calling. I had planned to visit Rethymnon and maybe the Palace at Knossos but perhaps I'll change my mind. I have no pressing schedule and tomorrow evening I set sail to Athens.

Christine and Kirstie leave today for England. We said our goodbyes last night. They certainly have been a comfort to me and an answer to my prayer. They have a very strong Christian Faith and Christine has shared her story, the abuse of her husband and subsequent divorce. I have found strength and healing through their essence. I shall miss them!

Since the sea is very calm today I decide to take advantage and swim in the late afternoon. It's far too hot to venture to the Palace at Knossos. I am content to read about this famous archaeological treasure and venture into Chania instead.

There are too many tourists milling about, but an adventure never the less. It's late when I return and therefore dinner is, too.

The usual fare: tomatoes, zucchini, cabbage, garlic, parsley, cucumbers and a potato this time. A glass of red wine and that's me

~ And So We Heal ~

finished for the day. I have a red heat rash on my lower legs that developed late evening. Not sure the cause but since so much of my body's purification is through my legs I accept it as detoxification. The moon time has finally ceased so I should be enjoying renewed vigour.

July 31, 2003 Delphi

The overnight ferry from Chania delivered me to Athens at six a.m. this morning. It was a wonderful experience onboard the 'Anek' ocean liner, sharing a cabin with two Greek ladies. Sitting outside on deck for hours staring up at the stars and out at the vast blackness all around, a gentle breeze touched my face and great gratitude welled up in my heart.

I was really proud of myself for making this journey- for 'pushing the boat out', and trusting that all would be taken care of.

When I eventually found the train station, that hooked me up to the wrong bus station from where I took the wrong bus, a taxi sped me to the correct bus station where I narrowly missed the early bus. Not to mind; three hours later and I was on my way.

Since I had not made reservations, arriving in Delphi I wandered around, somewhat delirious in the mid afternoon heat trying to find the perfect hotel at the perfect price. There are many, all with the names of the gods: The Apollo, and The Theseus, to name a few. It was the weight of my backpack that finally demanded I settle on something close at hand rather than wait for a messenger of the gods to whisper in my ear.

'The Artemis' it was then…. Sounded good to me and upon seeing that it had a balcony overlooking the rolling beauty, I was sold! The plumbing left something to be desired, but never mind. It's clean and following a long shower and a coffee enema, I'm remarkably refreshed

~ And So We Heal ~

and ready to go in search of sacred sites.

I wind my way down to the Temple of Athena and at the entrance find a beautiful bright green iridescent scarab beetle at my feet. I carefully wrap it up as some sort of auspicious treasure welcoming me to this magnificent site. It is absolutely awe inspiring – no other words. I spend almost two hours wandering around feeling the energy and fighting off the desire to dance wildly. Since there are people present I settle for taking lots of photos instead, but as the sun finally sets and I find myself alone there, I seize the moment and in a courageous dare to no one but myself, I bare my breasts.

It's close to ten when I wander into the liveliest taverna I can find and polish off a delicious omelette, Greek salad and a half carafe of homemade red wine. Alas, these legs of mine continue their purification, but other than my ankles burning, I feel no pain. It's the anniversary of Tom's death tomorrow and I shall visit Apollo.

On August 1st, the anniversary of Tom's death I would experience a miracle…

I was having dinner at a restaurant after visiting Apollo's temple when I met a stranger and his wife. I wrote the following piece about what happened:

BELIEVE

"Believe", said the stranger as he clasped his hands around mine.

I was speechless for once… caught in a whirlwind spinning me through the past few years of my remembering; spinning me back seven years to the day that Tom had died.

Perhaps misunderstanding my awestruck silence as doubt, his blue eyes grew big and passionate, his whole body perspiring in the humidity of the Greek summer evening.

"It doesn't matter if you don't believe", he continued…

~ And So We Heal ~

"It's ok, because I believe. I believe, I believe", he repeated; his voice growing more and more evangelistic...as if he was pulling the very words from my silence.

Finally, through the tears that were by now streaming down my smiling face.

"I DO BELIEVE...I do...I do!"

How could I possibly begin to tell this beautiful stranger all that was in my heart?

What amazing miracle was this that had brought me to Delphi to celebrate the seventh year since Tom had gone to heaven... Seven years to the very day! This was no coincidence. To be standing on this sacred ground with a complete stranger who when I had told him my story had asked nothing more than for me to BELIEVE, as he used his hands and his heart to 'take away my disease!' as he put it.

"I shall take it away, take it away!" he repeated, over and over, as he threw his body around a nearby tree.

And so it was that I left my 'breast cancer', (how I despise that word) with the gods and goddesses of Delphi.

Later that evening when the stranger was miles away I recalled his name as I lay in some beatific awe...Jon Francis...Tom's middle name was Francis...Thomas Francis...

BELIEVE...I hadn't just heard the word in that moment. I had actually seen it in big bold letters...right there in my third eye...just as it had appeared in the book I wrote *'Bridges a Memoir of Love'*. It was the last word on the last page, and it had come to mean everything to me over the years...

Seven years had passed since I had written that little book- it was time now to gather words again and shape them into another little book...

I BELIEVE...I STILL BELIEVE...

And I know that I always shall.

I shall always carry on believing...against all odds...I guess I was just born that way. I have seen so many miracles in my life over the years.

~ And So We Heal ~

We ultimately determine the quality of our lives, and I believe that disease can be cured by the mind, and its willingness to accept the miracle of life…

LOVE

August 8, 2003, UK

What an intense few days it's been. I return from my paradise feeling wonderful. My legs were swollen with the travelling and the altitude of the flight. They've never reduced that much since my long trek to Delphi but now several days later I can look at them and feel good. The right leg at the back of the knee feels a familiar ache and the lymph is swollen to the touch. I have a castor oil pack on it right now.

It was tough going to my three-month check up. I wasn't thinking too heavily upon the day. In the past it's been very stressful. Today I was fine up until twenty minutes before my consultation when I began to feel the usual unease..

Alison Waghorn, my consultant strode in with a wide smile and we set about the routine measuring of the lump. My blood tests came out fine and the cancer markers are normal but she tells me that these tests are not always reliable.

"Let's see how 'big' the lump is", she says

"How small!" I burst forth, determined to not let any negativity get to me.

She smiles, "It's bigger,"

I know that sometimes it feels that way, but I am not too bothered. The lower area again comes in for examination - dense - dimpling, p'eau d'orange. I've heard these words before.

I holdfast.

Truth is my breasts feel beautiful. They are brown and healthy looking from my time in Greece. I bared them at the Temple of Athena for God sake!

~ And So We Heal ~

A week ago I played the tambourine for Apollo at Delphi!

Words like core biopsy, Tamoxifen, Herceptin, return to the table. All words designed to change my state of being, but I'm not having any of it!

Later walking through the streets of Liverpool I try my best to shake it all off. I really like Alison a lot, and I know she has my best interests at heart, but these visits always take their toll. Returning home, my friend Jane calls to say her news was not good. She received the results from her bone and CT scan.

"The cancer has spread all over", she tells me...

Bones, ribs, parts of the lungs.

I am in shock. It doesn't seem possible. Poor Jane, she's fought so hard.

I realise I can only pray and hold the highest thoughts.

August 13, 2003, UK

We had a wonderful birthday party for mum at the caravan at the weekend. I am so grateful to have the love and support of my family. My sisters and I cycled up to Humphrey's Head, and on a dare we bared our naked breasts to the elements. It was so liberating that I stripped off and went romping through the green fields enjoying the freedom and abandonment especially with all the heaviness hanging over me.

Yesterday I rode the bus with a neighbour, Bernie. He's a man I often see walking with a cane, but rarely have the opportunity to talk to. Today was different – serendipity was at play. Our conversation revolved around health issues and he mentioned he'd had back surgery – two heart attacks and a stroke and on informing his doctor that he didn't feel good about taking too many pills the doctor told him he was depressed and prescribed anti-depressants. I told him I was going for acupuncture and somehow he got on to the subject of breast cancer, unaware of my condition. He actually quoted an article saying, far too many mastectomies were being performed and lumps needlessly removed. Now what are the odds of this conversation?

I knew that the gods were working their magic again.

Somehow I had plugged back in to the source of my healing and it came from within.

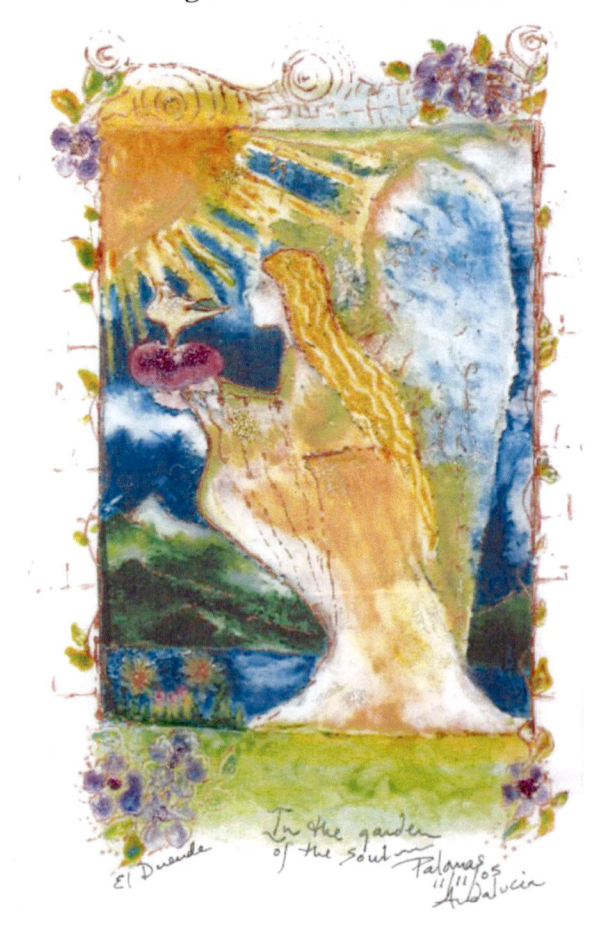

Chapter Ten
Here Comes the Light

As fate would have it, the Shumei Taiko drummers were invited to play at the Parliament of the Worlds Religions again, an event that has been taking place every five years since 1893. I had been the official Narrator for the group at the previous Parliament in Cape Town. It was now scheduled for Barcelona, and I had been asked to help co-ordinate Shumei's participation there.
Thinking back to the dreams I had had the last time I was in Barcelona, it all began to make sense.

There was one dream in which the lead drummer and Javier were making a circle around me, and another in Montserrat when I was being offered a drink of water by one of the ministers, each time a bell sounded. Both people concerned were scheduled to attend the event, and coincidentally, the theme of the Parliament was 'Water'. Coincidence?

It was in late 2000, if you remember, after I had just finished touring with the Shumei Taiko Ensemble when Javier had got back in touch. Destiny had brought me full circle, back to Spain then, and knowing how ill Javier was at the time I was grateful to have some role in his healing. Now it seems destiny was conspiring again to bring me back…

~ And So We Heal ~

October 26, 2003, Barcelona
Time passes quickly as always. It's two years, yesterday, since my diagnosis.

I have been on the move a lot lately. My journey to Crete and Delphi gave me extra confidence to continue on with my life.

Indeed I have ventured forward bravely, but it has not been without a struggle. Coming to Barcelona, almost two weeks ago now, re-united me with Javier. It had been ten months since my last visit. For the pre-opening ceremony of the parliament, I remember being seated in the Cathedral at Placa del Pi; camera in hand as was often the case, busy documenting the event. It was not until I stood to leave that I saw Javier. He had been sitting behind me all that time…

I realised later that it was no easy thing for him to sit still albeit in a church through such a long event.

As always it is a sweet joy to discover that we still both delight in each others presence, but inevitably the joy is accompanied by a pain which lets me know that there is still a ways to go with my emotional healing. But now with the acceptance and understanding of this pain as purification, hopefully I can traverse its peaks and valleys with more ease. Tears still fall, but they stop eventually and another part of who I am quickens and life becomes clearer.

Perhaps I will never understand what it is between us two, Javier and myself. I don't try to find those answers any more. My life must move forward. My light must continue to shine. There is still a lot of work to do. I pray simply that our relationship be blessed. That it be continuous, and nurture our spirits.

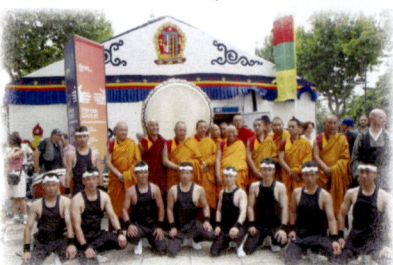

2004
I would spend most of the year 2004 involved with helping Shumei in Barcelona and continuing with

~ And So We Heal ~

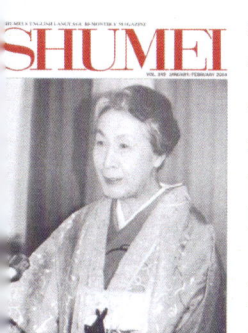

my own healing. I knew that the opportunity would be of great overall benefit to my well being on the one hand, and a good chance to further resolve the conflict with Javier, but I think that the stress of trying too hard to help others when I myself was still healing, ultimately took its toll.

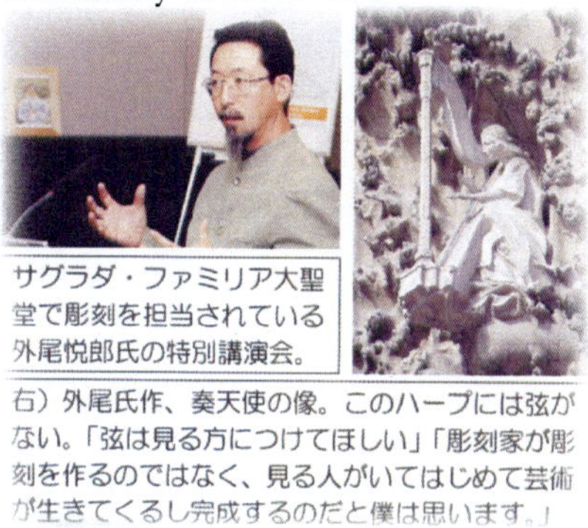

Perhaps I was a little too premature in thinking I could return so soon to 'normal' life when the truth was, so much revolved around my regime and getting enough rest. I wanted so much to inspire and be of service to others, but I had my limits.

The truth was, I still had this cancerous lump inside my breast and little did I know that the biggest challenge of all still lay ahead.

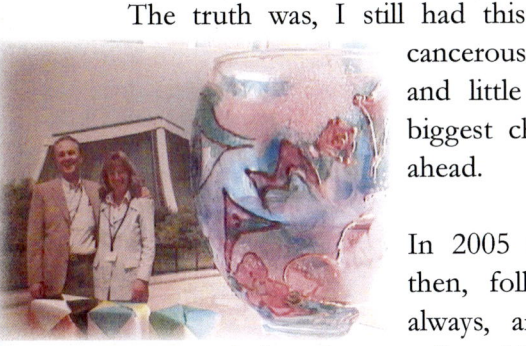

In 2005 the journey continued then, following my instinct as always, and investigating those recommendations that came from friends. Careful nutritional guidance is most important.

There is a goldmine of help if we are open to it...

My Sister, Deborah who owns the 'Rainforest' shop in Chester, with her partner Graeme, would write this about one of my adventures:

~ And So We Heal ~

February 9, 2005, UK

It's twelve O'clock, I'm thinking about this morning seeing Polly, (Pauline) off at the station. She's amazing my sis'; off she goes, with our parting war cry,

"Ya wander!"...Making me laugh as usual.

Shouldn't it be us raising her spirits, being positive and strong? But no, it's always her lifting us. I suddenly thought; you know what, I haven't been taking her visit to see the 'psychic surgeon' Steven Turroff, seriously enough! Maybe it wasn't going to be a case of HIM actually working this miracle; but that it was the actual journey, that she was taking; having to make such an effort with it...travelling down to London, lugging her big heavy case as always.

Maybe, the INTENT was the important thing. So I was compelled then to bring the family in to focus at the same time. I quickly called 'Edi', our mum. I didn't need to explain really, she knew what to do. Then I phoned Ann our sister-in-law. She sounded so good and before I'd even mentioned it she'd lit a candle, and wanted to know what time. We agreed on 12.30 and she'd call Michael our brother who was in Newcastle.

I left Graeme in the shop and went into the back room with my candle taking one of Polly's glass chalices, with the word 'Joy' on it'. I put a cushion on the floor and began a yoga breath to calm and focus myself. At first I was gazing at the chalice and imagining the letter 'o' in joy as a nipple, and trying to extract her tumour with my willpower; but I quickly stopped myself. It didn't feel right. So I just closed my eyes and emptied my mind... aware of my thoughts but not developing them.

A wave of peace came over me and then a familiar smell of 'old Holborn' tobacco, accompanied by a warm breath. It was my dad, who is deceased. (He seemed to be having a good time) Performing one of his magic tricks, where he would shove a hankie in his hand and make

~ And So We Heal ~

it disappear. He repeated it over and over again showing me his empty hand, saying,

"It's gone, it's gone. It's so simple" he said, with a beaming smile.

When I opened my eyes only fifteen minutes had gone by. I wasn't upset, although tears had rolled down my face. I just felt this incredible peace. I'm feeling more emotional now as I recall it. But at the time, I didn't try to cling to him, and I wasn't sad to open my eyes. I just wanted to speak to Pauline to try to convey the beaming image of Pa saying, "It's so simple…it's gone, it's gone"

Can it really be that simple?

So now you know…it runs in the family! God Bless my sister Debbie.

It's gone, it's gone! became my mantra from then on, and very nearly the title of this book. I had always looked upon my healing as an 'alchemical process' of purification.

The alchemists believed that by working with the forces of alchemy, anyone could not only tap into hidden sources of creative power, but could fundamentally transform themselves and their life situations. There were seven stages in alchemy and not always in a specific order – calcination, dissolution, separation, conjunction, fermentation, distillation, and coagulation.

In my case I seem to have begun with calcination in 2001 around the time of my diagnosis…

'…During this a person must endure the most horrendous hell-fire that eventually reduces ones life to shambles (it involves working with fire to burn away mental constructs and reveal a persons true essence.')

In 2005, on February 19th, my friend Jane Lawn Redmond finally lost her long heroic battle and died.

I was away at the time and her death affected me deeply. She had always been so resilient. I began to question where exactly I was in this seemingly never-ending 'purification'. I would often delve into my diaries and writings from the past to find the clues to the future.

Finding this written in an envelope tucked behind a watercolour I painted of 'Isis', put me back on track:

December 2nd 2001, El Duende, Andalucia

…My birthday… I have followed a calling, if you will, to the hills of Andaluia. I came here to heal my soul…my mind…my physical body. I am carrying a lump in my right breast, close to my heart chakra. I know without a doubt that this 'hardening', is connected to my emotional journey…to my loving heart that has been taking quite a beating. I recognise what this healing must embrace.

Instinctively, I seem to be reaching for those things that will nourish me…body, mind and spirit. It is not enough for me to simply agree to the surgery that will only remove a symptom and then brutally saturate my being with toxic chemicals and fire radiation at my tissues with the hopes that all this may stop the invaders. It is my essence that speaks most clearly to me now…my truth believes that-

'First ye shall do no harm'

It is not an easy path, this one…Great pain, and great loss, great suffering, yes…
But I know without a doubt…this too shall pass, as if in a dream…
   These tears that pour from somewhere deep within, are tears of purification…

~ And So We Heal ~

Through them the light of transformation gives new birth…Today is my birthday. I am 50 years old. Four months ago I had no idea that my birthday would be spent high in the hills of Andalucia, with tinkling goat bells, and voices echoing through the mountains.

All is a stranger to me here,
And yet in truth,
'All' is part of the 'one thing'.

As always, my story is about Love…It is about following ones heart, and believing in a dream. I came here to Spain to make a decision. To live…Simply to Live!

My sacrifice would be to release the fears that bind, let go of expectations, and believe without a doubt that my pain would be healed, all in good time.

I am here to breathe in the energy of Light
To exhale the sorrows of a lifetime…
To re-commit myself to loving,
And to calling back my spirit…

'All is part of the 'ONE THING.'

There it was again, like a 'wake-up' call. I always seemed to find it within my very own notes. Once again I opened up the book *The Emerald Tablet* by, Dennis William Hauck to find:

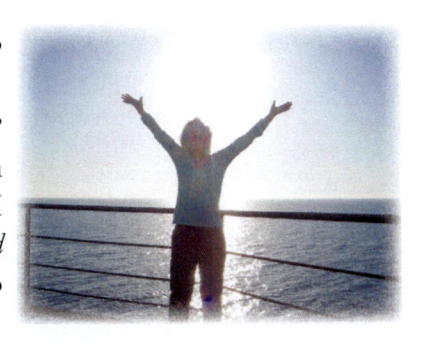

…The alchemists whose craft was both spiritual and material in nature, actually developed step-by-step procedures for working in a rarefied realm and learning to alter reality, over the centuries discovering ways of accessing the One mind, and transmuting physical and spiritual elements through the 'One Thing'. Over the last two millennia alchemists have written millions of words trying to describe the 'One thing'. It all seemed to lead back to the ancient dictum-

'Know thyself'

That was the message I had encountered in Delphi.

Over three years had passed since I journeyed through those first years following my diagnosis. I had come to Barcelona wanting to help save Javier's life, and in the process nearly lost my own. I was beginning to think that somewhere along the way I had given my power away. Just when I thought I knew myself, I felt as if I was being tested yet again...

May 29, 2005, UK
I awake this morning feeling very alone. I've been trying to push forward with this book but it is taking all my strength to just get through each day. I am on my period so I know it is connected to my hormones. Tears are falling and I imagine all sorts of things. I am lost again. Something is eating away at my heart.

As I inch my way through the typing up of my diaries for the last several years, I take this time to try to express all that I have been going through.

It started with my return to Barcelona from England in 2004, and the news that Javier has had more angina pains. I knew something was happening. I had felt it within my own body- in unison- the physical, and emotional.

In August the same year I had tried 'Compound X' paste after studying about the use of various salves for extracting tumours. Ingrid Naiman's book, 'Salves that Heal' (See appendix) is very informative

~ And So We Heal ~

on the subject. At the time I felt that the tumour wanted to be drawn out through the skin. After reading some of the documentation going back to the early 1800's, I found doctors who were using salves successfully back then and many success stories on various sites on the internet. I had great faith in this process, but I really needed a nurse to help with the dressing. It was an extremely hot summer and what started as a test patch with the salve, ended by it melting and burning little holes on my breast. All of this was happening as the 'Parliament' began to get underway…I was extremely busy but trying to keep to my regime. The Shumei taiko drummers had arrived and we had arranged for them to give a concert in Lleida, which was very successful but the day took its toll on me. With the hot summer heat the wounds began to turn nasty and suppurate. I panicked and chose to stop the process, something they warn against doing.

The search was on then to find a solution to the apparent mess I'd made of things, although I always try to maintain that **everything** happens for a reason. An assortment of continuous poultices, including green clay, castor oil and turmeric, with dressings being changed twice a day, helped a little and of course my mantra – **It's Gone!!!**

The truth is …I am undergoing some heavy emotional cleansing that I relate to the tumour preparing to leave my body…I get regular hands-on healing from Jose Antonio, the wonderful faith healer I have been seeing for the past year in Barcelona. He has an amazing story. After experiencing major head pain that would come and go he one day collapsed and fell under a train. He was in a coma for ninety days during which time his wife left him and they amputated his leg. When he came out of the coma his stomach had ninety percent cancer, but he somehow survived to awaken to his own gifts as a healer. Seeing him always makes me feel strong and hopeful. Sometimes when he is working on me I feel intense heat and flashes of purple light.

I've been taking Carctol, the ayurvedic herbs championed by Dr. Rosy Daniel, at the Bristol Centre (now the Penny Brohn Centre) It's been three months almost, and although I don't feel any shrinkage, the sheer necessity to drink three litres of water a day has done me good.

At the moment I am researching something called 'ECT, Electrochemical tumour therapy in Malaga that although expensive seems to be beckoning me. I will use my credit card, and slowly pay it off.

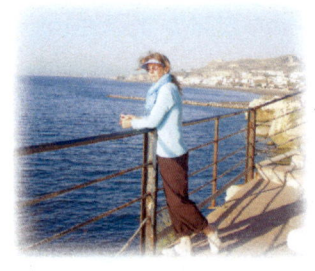

Something is calling me back to Andalucia. It will be good to go back again after almost four years. I can always fly back to Barcelona if Javier needs me. At the moment he is building up his strength again after the last angina attack. We both need to take more care of ourselves.

'The Alchemist', Paul Coelho:
Fatima to shepherd boy, "the desert takes our men from us, and they don't always return. We know that, and we are used to it. Those who don't return become a part of the clouds, a part of the animals that hide in the ravines, and of the water that comes from the earth. They become part of everything - they become the soul of the world".

June 5, 2005, Barcelona
Slept well…although feeling a little out of sorts. I am more determined than ever to release all the negativity out of each cell in the body and proceed in the light.

I awake this morning with images of frogs in my dreams…LEAPING… and also the name of Dr. Ryke Geerd Hamer appears…

It's a powerful omen to me to acknowledge that I am on the right path. As I mentioned previously I have been tremendously impressed by his work and believe fully in his theory known as 'German New Medicine':

~ *And So We Heal* ~

After twenty years of research and therapy with over 31,000 patients, Dr. Hamer finally established firmly, logically and empirically how biological conflict – shock results in a cold cancerous or necrotic phase, and how, if the conflict is resolved, the cancerous or necrotic process is reversed to repair the damage and return the individual to health.

For the rest of the day I explore my emotions…
The winds of change are upon me.
Separation is inevitable.

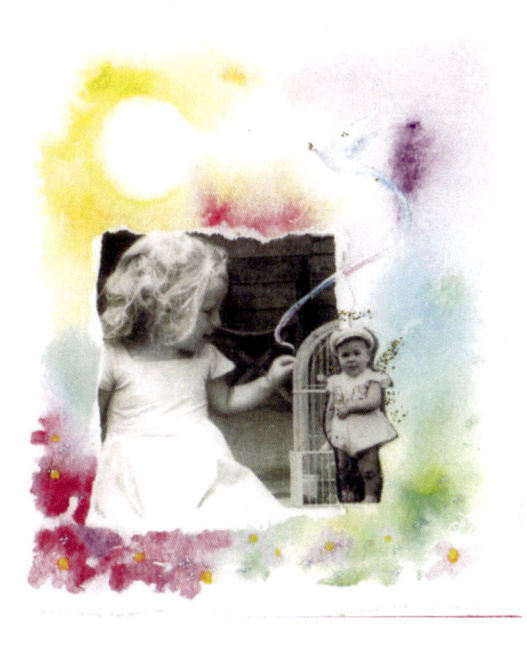

I know Javier is suffering with his health and when he is unwell his emotions affect mine. We have become so close over these last years that sometimes I feel 'his' childhood hurts and in an effort to try to nurture him I find myself smothering him. I know the dark side of him is in control when he tells me that there is no future to our story…

~ And So We Heal ~

An inner 'courageous self' urges me to hold fast...to not be bitter.
It is a dark night of the soul...
But I fight to remain disconnected,
To pray as always to keep us in the light.
To understand...
To communicate...
And to love

A whispered presence urges me to master the emotions...and wake rejuvenated in the morning ready for the next stage...

The frogs in my dream came to signal ...

SUCCESS...

LEAPING FORWARD...
Transformation and friendship...

I know I must bear this again...
The difference is ...

I AM DIFFERENT
I AM STRONGER
I THUS SURVIVE

June 13, 2005, Barcelona

Set my alarm for six but am awake at five a.m...lying there listening to my own stressful breathing. This morning I have an appointment with a Spanish oncologist at Hospital San Pau.

My Spanish friend Marian Mateos whom I met through the Parliament last year, has insisted that she come with me. She is a real gem, an auxiliary nurse's aid. The oncologist is a young woman, a child almost in my eyes…or is it that I am old? She has the usual stern look of death upon her face when I tell her that I do not want chemotherapy or radiation. Finally she goes to get her senior, and although they both mean well they serve up the usual scare tactics, and utter amazement as to why I have not received the so called normal – (I'll be crass here) cut, poison, and burn treatment up until now. They were essentially pointing a finger at me and saying if you do not do this, that, and the other you WILL DIE!!!

God knows I try to stay calm, but when it's my life that they are discussing, I cannot hold back.

"Heyyyyyyyyy now!!!!" I'm on my feet with a familiar 'Thelma and Louise' battle cry.

"My life is MY LIFE…and I decide what I will and will not do with It"…on and on I rant… all in Spanish - and not that bad if I may say so, but thank God for dear Marian, on hand to buffer the awkward moments and fill in the missing words as they bounce off the walls.

This is Hollywood award time people!

I mean all I actually want are some bloody blood tests and perhaps a 'pet scan'. But nothing doing - In the end I am sent back to a GP to order them. It's my bad luck to get another practitioner who once again stares at me with a death sentence.

"Do you know anybody who has survived advanced breast cancer?" she asks.

"YES… YES…AND YES!!!!!!!"

Of course she's not buying any of it, but reluctantly orders the blood tests, all the while talking to me like I am 'dead woman walking.'

Oh the horror of it all…by the time I navigate the polluted streets of Barcelona and make it back, I am well and truly wiped out. My breasts feel like melons again, and there is a negative cloud just waiting to rain down on me. A quick stop at the Internet café in the hopes that I can find some words of wisdom to cheer me on, but …nada!! I trudge along then through the final alley thinking that the 'angels', had all taken the day off, when there it was…the messenger of good tidings, Jordi Griera, Marian's partner, on the phone. He's calling from a car ambling through the French countryside. Marian has obviously spoken to him about what the Oscar-worthy scene she witnessed this morning at the hospital.

God bless these two!

"What were you doing at the hospital anyway?" he asks.

"Don't you know that they are there to scare the hell out of you?"

Jordi's English is perfect. Of course he was being a little facetious but his words serve to uplift me immediately. They all mean well – hopefully! They are only doing their job. Jordi continues on quoting me a very potent passage of the 'Bhagavad-Gita.'

The telephone connection is not the best, but with those words I do hear…'fire…hunger…food…Brahma…being the god of one's own life'….drifting in from the French countryside, I am lifted from the potential depths…the possible fray. I am able to fight on! Tears spring from my eyes…gratefully so. This is no time to bottle anything up… I must move forward…ULTREYA…

~ And So We Heal ~

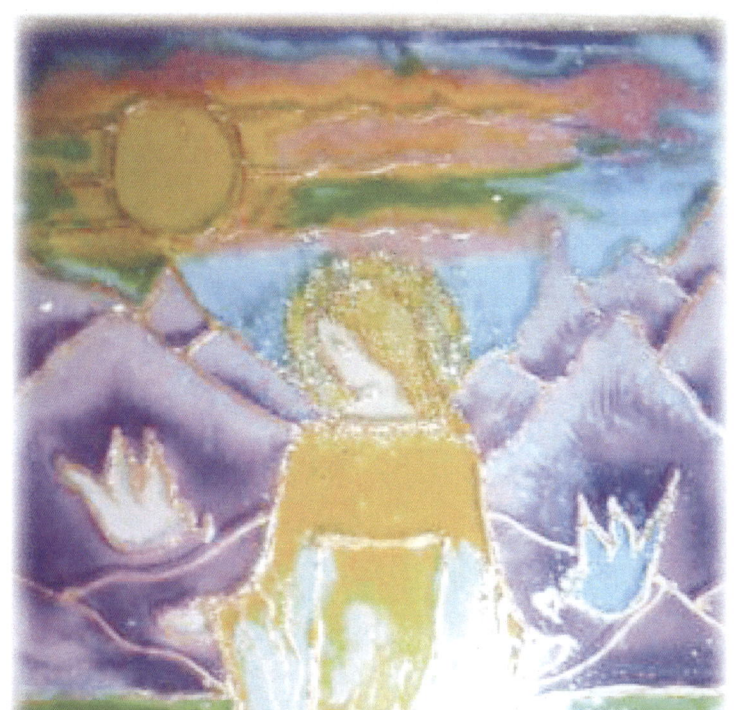

Later as I reach for one of Rumi's poems, I find…
In any gathering
In any chance meeting on the street, there is a shine, an elegance rising up!
Today I recognised that the jewel-like beauty is the presence, our loving confusion, the glow in which watery clay gets brighter than fire, the one we call friend. I begged, "Is there a way into you; a ladder?"
"Your head is the ladder; bring it down under your feet. The mind, this globe of awareness is a starry universe that when you push off with your foot, a thousand new roads become clear. As you yourself do at dawn, sailing through the light."

RUMI

June 15, 2005, Barcelona

I awoke from a beautiful dream in which I had found a blue iridescent bird in the bushes. It stepped gently into my hand. I was absolutely captivated by this treasure...

Then somehow the dream had me sliding along, and when I stood up my thigh was icy and wet...a foreboding that my newfound joy would come at a price as always.

June 17, 2005, Barcelona

As I lay drifting off to sleep during a siesta the image of a water faucet with water running on to a small bowl of broken glass...then my finger is burnt as I light the boiler...Fire and Water!!

Fire...Mmmmm......I wonder!

I open up 'The Emerald tablet' again and choosing a page at random am led to read about Mercury. The alchemists talk about a 'secret fire' that quickens the soul - associated with the process of 'fermentation' in which new life is brought to dead and decaying matter. During this stage one enters into quietness to connect with the higher mind in order to transform and quicken ones being as it is this higher consciousness- the thoughts from above that enlighten us.

However, before this comes 'Putrefaction': 'dark night of the soul'. This calls for the absolute suppression of ego, which is an indispensable requirement for moving into a higher dimension of consciousness from dark depression.

The alchemist must forbear during this uncomfortable phase of lost identity, while the base elements within transmute into nobler elements, and into the next stage known as 'Quintessence'.

I spend the rest of the day trying to arrange for my treatment in Malaga. Since the summer solstice is next week my intuition is pushing for then. It will be a bit of a rush, but the idea of having this during the 'fire' celebrations appeals to me. It's the perfect chance to burn off the dross, so to speak.

Chapter Eleven

El Duende

> El Duende is the passion, and the quickening.
> El Duende is the lover and the lovemaking and the life born from the lovemaking. It is everything. How does it choose whom to descend upon? Aye, it comes to the one who has laid out food for it, the one who has left the door open for it, the one who yearns for such a quest...
>
> Women Who Run With Wolves

June 23, 2005, Malaga,

I arrived in Malaga yesterday to a heat wave. As part of the annual summer solstice; St John's day in Spain, with its purification rites, there are fires burning all over Spain, and the biggest full moon in eighteen years. Good God is this auspicious timing or what??

Having seriously debated my next step of healing the 'tumour', I elected to come to Malaga and meet with Laurent Schidler, at the 'Medibio Clinic'. (See appendix p126) We've been communicating via email:

As a naturopath, he is using an electrotherapy device, BET / ECT, and a 'PAPIMI', machine, amongst other things.

~ And So We Heal ~

ELECTRONIC THERAPIES: Rife, Beck, Clark, and others have used electronic therapies to treat cancer. Many have had successes treating cancer using these devices.
Electrotherapy, also known as electrochemical tumor therapy, Galvanotherapie and electro-cancer treatment (ECT), was developed in Europe by the Swedish professor Björn Nordenström and the Austrian doctor Rudolf Pekar. The therapy employs galvanic electrical stimulation to treat tumors and skin cancers. ECT is used most often as an adjunct with other therapies. Using local anesthesia, the physician inserts a positively-charged platinum, gold or silver needle into the tumor and places negatively-charged needles around the tumor. Voltages of 6 to 15 volts are used, dependent upon tumor size.

My research and intuition have led me here. His communication with me, thus far over the telephone, has been very positive, although I am still a little confused as to exactly what treatment I should choose.

Meeting with Laurent and his doctor in residence, Doctora M. Eudoxia Lopez Peral, was a very powerful experience on many levels. Walking into the clinic, with its calming blue light, soft music, and fragrance wafting through the air I was immediately put at ease. We discussed my case history, and they were impressed with all that I was doing thus far as part of trying to strengthen my immune system to fight the disease.

Laurent's wife, Simone had had breast cancer ten years ago, and after traditional chemotherapy and radiation, the cancer recurred. He was a businessman at the time, but dropped everything, and devoted his life to finding an alternative treatment to save his wife's life. They found the ECT being used in China, and other European countries and it cured her cancer and so he decided to change fields and became a naturopath and scientific investigator.

~ And So We Heal ~

Doctora Marie Eudoxia, with the face of an angel struck me as being a very caring and compassionate soul...It helps that she also happens to be a homeopath as well as a top surgeon in her field. When she made reference to Saint Germaine, a famous alchemist, I felt 'goose bumps', as just the day before I had received a treatment from someone who worked with his trademark 'violet flame of transmutation', and I myself felt his presence, having for a long time worked with the energy of ascended masters, in my art.

I was to put my trust in these people...

It was as simple as that. Later as they examined me, I noticed that she carefully held her hand over the silver angel I wear around my neck, and my breast felt safe.

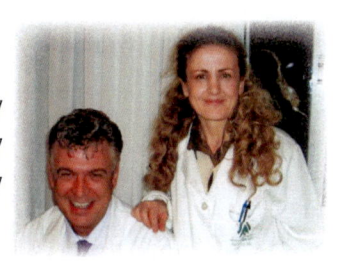

Thinking back to the time preceding this meeting, I remember that the tumour had been rapidly changing over the last weeks definitely attached to my emotional well-being....I just needed to be mindful, and watch for the signs along the way.

I had trusted that each step of my journey was being aided by a higher source, a collective force...

This was the key to my well being.

Reflecting on our conversation, I remember them asking if I had identified any apparent purpose to me growing this tumour...
   Dios mio!! What a question – where does one begin?
   I recounted my experience with the 'compound X' paste that I used the year before, when I was desperately trying to evict the tumour from my body. It was during the mid July heat, and the paste which was only

~ *And So We Heal* ~

meant to provoke a small opening, somehow melted and caused serious wounds to my breast. Staring at my breast in the mirror that night the scars formed the face of a new-born baby, and as I cupped it tenderly in my hands, once more the pain of silent screams and hot tears flooded through me as a reminder of the weight that I was in some way still carrying - 'The child that was never born'.

There is a theory I read in a book by Barbara Stone - 'Cancer as Initiation.' She quotes Russell Lockhart saying that "cancer is related to denying something in oneself - something of one's psychic and bodily earth, not allowed to live, not allowed to grow. Cancer lives something of life unlived."
I am more convinced than ever that in my case this is true!

Here I was again facing the remnants of broken dreams buried deep in my being and most surely connected to my dear Javier whose own blockages and heart problems I had willingly absorbed into my psyche. We had reached 'crisis point'.
It was time now to burn away all the past pain and hurt…all the lost dreams.
I stand straight now in front of the mirror, and hear myself say out aloud,

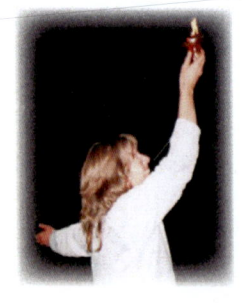

"I willingly release this 'stone',
this 'treasure' that has served me well,
Even as it came to take me to the edge of death.
I stand firm with my faith
and in refusing to stop loving,
I am re-born."

(**What?** - You think I was going to let all that dramatic theatrical training go to waste!)

~ *And So We Heal* ~

It's almost nine pm when I leave the hotel to take a walk along the beach. I'm hoping to see the many fires that will burn through the night, but it's still light out and they are just beginning. Today marks a big fiesta but the only flames I can find are those that are being stoked for the local skewered sardines, which have been calling to me. Strange how they called to me three and a half years ago up at 'El Duende'. It's all so symbolic being back in Andalucia at this time as I prepare to release my illness.

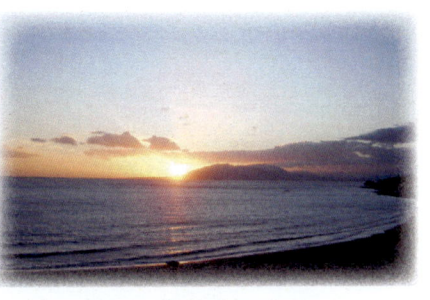

The journey has brought me full circle and enriched my life beyond imagining. I find the last rays of the golden sun to bask in at the local 'chiringuito' on the beach, and order a plate of fresh sardines I've just watched being roasted over the flames. The tiny glass of tinto warms my heart and I am fortified for what lies ahead.

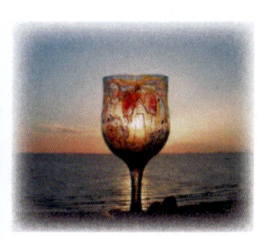

The next morning I arrive at the clinic for the first of what would be many sessions.

Soft music helped me to try to relax into the experience and forget about the reality of it all, as the doctors pierced the pertinent needles connected to electrodes in various positions in and around the tumour. Since I had a local anaesetic in the breast I could feel very little during this procedure, and preferred not to look as the mere thought of it was painful to my senses. The team were very gracious in their manner and worked well together, so I was able to give them my trust. They had never worked with a tumour this size before so no one could surmise exactly how many treatments I would need, but I was in it for the duration. There would be no turning back. Still, being only human after all I must admit to it being quite an ordeal, both physically and emotionally. I had opted only for a saline drip and minimal pain relief...perhaps now in retrospect I would have chosen to be 'put under' for the duration.

~ And So We Heal ~

In short, there was more physical pain than I had anticipated, accompanied by strong emotional waves as I recalled a lot of the pain in my life over the years. I sensed so many of my ancestors, friends and family who had passed on...they were all around the bed, together with images of others still alive today-my beloved support team in essence.

When all the needles were in place...six or seven, I believe; they fired up the voltage, which was then monitored on a computer screen. Almost immediately I could feel sharp stabs of electricity build to intensity, and pass through my breasts in waves. In my minds eye soft swirling colours of purple, yellow, blue, and pink came to pervade my senses, and it was through these that I searched for portals to other worlds...to anything really that could explain to me why it was necessary for me to be healed in this particular way.

'Had I been abducted after all?'

'Were these strange yet friendly aliens probing my psyche in order to advance their understanding of the female species?'

It was all quite surreal and not entirely unpleasant until about midway through when the colours were fading; I suddenly found myself in a greyish dense essence similar to that which I encountered when I came through my abortion. I became very emotional and Laurent held my hand and tried to help me relax. I began blowing air out in short bursts as if I was in labour. He actually likened the process to giving birth, as we were after all trying to induce the expelling of this large mass growing inside me.

'Good God...Just when you think you've laid the ghosts to rest!!!'

But this was no beautiful child inside me...it was the hardened detrius of all my broken dreams. Finally, after all these years I could come face to face with it.

"You've got to kick it out now", Laurent told me.

"You must be firm and tell it to leave. Think of it as Mr. Bush!!" he said, making me smile, but good God he had a point! After more than four years of carrying this around with me I had almost allowed it to become an accepted part of who I am. It was not going to give up without a fight! But neither was I?

If I was going to survive, (and I was) I truly had to get tough.

Back to being Lady Macbeth then…as inside my soul I told myself firmly:

"WITH THIS RELEASE I AM GIVING BIRTH TO MY SELF…
MY NEW SELF."

Almost immediately, I saw a small black dot in my third eye, and I remembered seeing the same thing many years ago during a meditation, and it scared me a little. It was, I thought, a premonition of some dark cloud that I would need to confront down the line. I never ever dreamed that it would be 'breast cancer'. (Funny how I can actually write these words now. I do so only in reference to the name of a so-called disease. I've never really believed that I had breast cancer, and now, less than ever.)

This is the key.

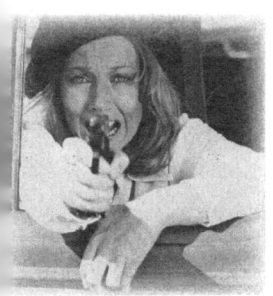

As the darkness descends I allow tears to fall and at one point hear myself say out loud,
   "Get behind me Satan."
   I say it with full conviction too, having used it often in the past whenever I thought that dark forces were at play and I needed protection.

~ And So We Heal ~

The abortion issue surfaces, but not with any grand degree of emotion…more of a light memory when a metal door seemed to slam shut on some part of my life. It was the same door that slammed upon hearing the news of Tom's death.

It is without any shadow of doubt that I recognise the role that shock and grief have played in my dis-ease.

Without any fanfare the angels appear then to pull on this mass that has surely begun it's demise. There are two of them hauling up what appears to be a dark ectoplasm of sorts.

The black spot disappears and when the pain gets a little too much La Doctora is there to lower the voltage, hold my hand and affect some gentle change to my distressed state. I glance at the clock and see that there is still one more hour to go.

How can I possibly endure, I wonder, when she whispers in my ear, "*Quatro minutos*, four minutes…"

No me digas…Dios mio! - My God!" my elated response.

I can hardly believe it. I am battle weary, and disoriented a little from the medication that I'm not used to, but I'm on my feet. The journey has really just begun.

June 30, 2005, Andalucia

Last nights dream: I was beside an iron gate, and up to my waist in water that was steadily rising. My thoughts were that if I could only snap the curling iron I could squeeze my body through and swim out somehow. I asked where everybody else was and a voice came to tell me that they were just lying down somewhere...accepting what was coming. There seemed to be a feeling of impending doom, and I was desperately trying to get my head through the gate but it was no use...then suddenly at the moment I decided to fight, a door behind me opened and the waters abated. It was almost like a miracle, and the fact that I had decided to take firm action was the key.

It's strange…I had completely forgotten about the dream until the word 'hierro', meaning 'iron' in Spanish seemed to jump out at me from a cereal box that morning.

Later in the day I walked up to the spring to get water. My body was feeling very stiff after yesterday's treatment, so I moved quite gingerly. Just as I approached the well, I started to cry remembering that towards the end of the treatment I suddenly had a vision of the 9/11 disaster in America with people jumping to their deaths from the Twin Towers. I was in California at the time and had seen it all live on television. Since I was in a very low emotional state anyway because of losing contact with Javier, I've often wondered if perhaps feeling vulnerable at the time, my psyche had recorded some of the horror of the victims. They do say that after 9/11 there was an increase in cancer in America.

I'm reminded of a dream I had shortly after my diagnosis in which I was clutching an American flag to my right breast.

Yesterday's treatment was quite intense as they put an extra needle through the top of my breast. The pain came in undulating waves; the idea of it all perhaps being the hardest to bear. I spent the time chanting to myself…God – light, love…all the positive words I could muster. When the energy was bearable the colours were definitely healing. At one point I also felt the presence of my aunt Maisie who had died of uterine cancer. She seemed to be exuding a silent strength and assured me that I was doing the right thing. She herself was subjected to the horrors of radium.

It would take at least four sessions before a crust began to appear on the surface of my breast signalling that the necrosis was pushing its way out. Since I was not living in Andalucia I could not complete the process in one go and elected to keep returning to Malaga over a period of eighteen months or so.

Once again it is my diaries that help me keep track of what would turn out to be quite an amazing experience, to say the least. About five months into the treatment I experience a breakthrough.

November 17, 2005, Andalucia

I had another ECT treatment a few days ago-with the usual tiredness after, and expelling a lot of liquid-this time brown toffee-like looking stuff with an awful odour. I bear with it all and concentrate on building up my strength.

Yesterday I walked up the mountain to Comares. I had not the usual 'steam in my engine' for such a trek, but I did it nonetheless, taking the high road up through rugged terrain…huffing and puffing along… quite breathless really when my own audible gasp nearly sent me off balance. There in the bushes was the torso of what appeared to be a goat. After a lengthy, earnest pause, I managed to move past squeamishness in order to examine the carcass (from a distance of course) to see if it held any specific significance for me. Finding none apparently, I continued walking until I came across a whole pen of goats staring down at me...our communication as always in awed silence.

As a treat I stop at a local restaurant and have my favourite two fried eggs and lovely toast and butter, and a glass of de-caf. Since I only had fruit this morning I'm quite ravenous. It's nice to sit and read the local paper. An old re-run of 'Bonanza', is playing on the television. My God...nothing's changed. It was the same thirty-six years ago when I lived in Spain. I lose myself in a time warp of my own comforts and get very little writing done. Still, I remind myself, this part of the journey is not about writing. It's about recuperating. Let's face it, it's taking a lot to move this mass out of my body In the afternoon I do a little painting. The crystal chandelier droppers I bought in Florence are calling to me, and before I know it the angels are back...almost effortlessly, I notice. They seem to know who they are. Archangel Michael is the most forthcoming, his strong blue cape always first to be painted.

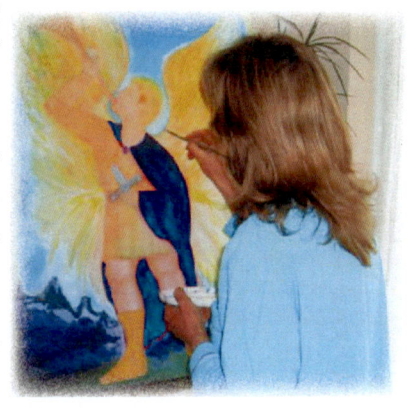

Physically there is an ongoing pain that is just about tolerated. It doesn't warrant using prescription medicine, so I continue with the Traumeel-homeopathic meds.

The sun disappears early these days and by five pm, my energy is a little drained. I don't have much appetite apart from hot soupy broth with cayenne and ginger. By nine I am ready for bed. The pain is droning on and I keep a hot water bottle with me at all times. The body seems to want to just lie down and manage the pain.

~ *And So We Heal* ~

My friend Helen calls from England and I am glad to catch up on things with her. Our friend Denise has not been too well, and has hit a crisis-point with her own ongoing battle with breast cancer. We discuss options for her and the issue of pain management. I thank God, have had such minimal pain it would seem. Case in point, by the time I hang up, the pain has subsided. Just taking my mind off it, helped actually.

Before bed I decide to change my dressings again. There has been little discharge today and I am disappointed as there is still a lot to break down yet.

However, this time as I remove the swabs I am met with enormous discharge, foul smelling stuff, and a piece of tissue seems to be dangling from my breast.

"Oh my God"...I am in a sudden state of shock.

"What the he- - is it?"

"Oh my God, Oh my God...could it be the nipple??"

The precious nipple that I have fought so hard to save. It's been slowly burying itself lately. I had asked Laurent on Monday if he thought I would lose it, and he felt that it was most probable, since the tumour was now directly behind it. I had to face up to the awful reality now, as I scrambled then to open a new pack of swabs whilst holding wads of cotton over the wound.

Hot liquid pours out as I stand up, and I feel it splash onto my white sock...eeeeeeeeeeehhhh!!...I am now on my tip toes, dancing around in childish squealing...whilst in a constant dialogue with the almighty.

"Heavenly Father, Mother, Goddess, Madonna!...You name it...I beseeched them all. The Lord's Prayer spills out over and over again reminding me of the first few months after my diagnosis when I would repeat it three times daily. What a strange experience it all was... scary but exciting at the same time. Almost too much to deal with at this moment so I manage to wrap the breast up well, and bundle myself into bed where I lay in silence with my hand gently cupped around the wounded 'creature'. The main pain has disappeared, replaced now with a tingling sensation and an odd hollowness, a black hole in my psyche. All I can think is - this used to be my breast…all those fine capillaries scooped out now…decaying flesh returning to the earth as it were.

Finally, the thing that I had been praying for over these long four years. Finally I was experiencing results. But it was only just beginning, I had to be really strong now and, in Laurent's words, 'Kick the bastard out!' But it was not so easy; this was after all my breast. There was still some good tissue involved. I reach over and caress the other breast. It feels soft and perfect. I've always thought I had a pretty lovely pair of breasts. That reality really does not exist for me now. I lay there in the candlelight, reviewing 'who I am now'.

How much further will this healing journey take me?

I had called down the gods on Monday during my treatment. In my visualization I had felt the thrust of Archangel Michael's sword until I almost fainted, chanting over and over,

"I am cancer-free, I am cancer-free!"

I had begged God to be swift with this stage of it all-thinking that I could not possibly bear so much pain anymore, and now, here it was, the fruit of all that suffering.

Waking up around 1.30 a.m. to change the dressing again I find it is sopping wet with the familiar brown fudge. The dangling tissue breaks off now effortlessly, and I wrap it up quickly, hardly able to acknowledge what it might be. I'll deal with it in the morning. I do manage to sleep some more and am awake by seven forty five am in time to see Ruth driving off for her yoga class in Competa. If all had progressed as hoped, I would have gone with her but today is one of those days that calls for complete and utter rest.

~ And So We Heal ~

Now as I reflect on last night's drama I perceive it all as a giving birth of sorts. The tissue that came off is still carefully wrapped up. I somehow find the courage to peep at it and in doing so am reminded of the day my mother brought my newborn sister Debbie home from the hospital, and I found her detached and shrivelled umbilical cord wrapped up in tissue. How strange is life. This whole ordeal is like 'the giving birth' I never got to experience. There is still a measure of pain with me, yes. But the truth is that I am a new being today...

There is a stronger light within me now.

November 19, 2005, Andalucia

Saturday morning here at 'El Duende'. I awake from the usual deepest of sleeps around 8.00 a.m. Yoga is at 10 - but my body is telling me to sit this one out. The hole in the breast is still weeping out debris. It's a honey coloured liquid now with lots of black carbon lumps. The whole mass seems to have reduced considerably and I am so very grateful for this inner strength that I have to do battle with. There is intermittent sharp needle type pain, but nothing that I cannot handle. I try to keep the right side flexible. The shoulders are so tense where I am over compensating to protect myself.

The horror of the other night has abated now and I seek to fill the emptiness of the open wound with a soft love. I can definitely feel that a big part of the tumour has died. I feel lighter and almost dreamlike in the knowledge and experience of it all. My period has been quite heavy so this is definitely a time of releasing 'stuff'.

In lieu of yoga I walk up to the spring to fill my water bottles. Moving slowly feels good; but on examination of my mind I feel that I am carrying thoughts about so many of my friends. My mind is rarely inactive, always thinking of others, always full of creativity.

Finally it seems, I am beginning to accept and understand the true meaning of El duende in my life:

The spirit, the immense spirit, often misunderstood as a force of all that is, all that will ever be…Espiritu Sanctu, Pisces Sophia or Ruach, – the breath of God- Hagia Sophia, "wind of knowing". It is said that 'El Duende' can split a person's heart and mind wide open, that it can descend to inspire a person, to shake or impregnate a person or to put something into a person that they have been emptied of or that they have never had before, like grace for instance.

January 15, 2006, Andalucia

My dream: I am standing upright on my mother's shoulders with my arms outstretched, victorious. An unidentified male walks beside us.

My dear mother has been such a loving support to me over the years - as have all my family and friends.

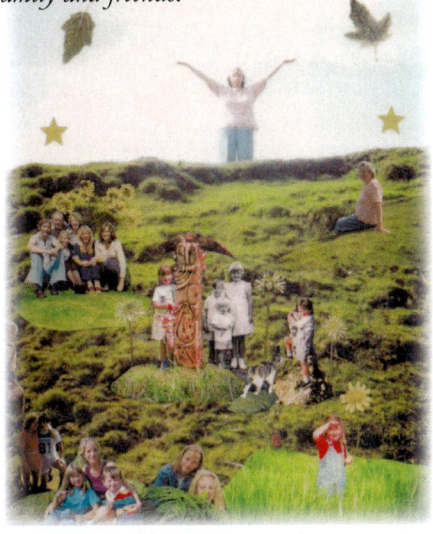

~ *And So We Heal* ~

I left Barcelona three days ago on the early morning flight to Malaga. My ECT treatment was scheduled for ten o'clock. A few days before, I began to experience the usual nervousness about the procedure so I decided that regardless of what the results were, this would be my last ECT, making it the tenth. My breast, or rather what was left of it, seemed to be letting me know that the hard fight was pretty much over; although I was still dressing it twice a day, as the necrosis would still take time to fully evacuate my body.

Arriving from the airport at Malaga bus station with thirty minutes to spare before my appointment I sat on a bench to bask in the early morning sunshine somehow managing to finish off the oatmeal and yoghurt I'd brought with me to line my stomach against the usual 'diazepam' I'd grown accustomed to. Forgetting a spoon made it a messy job, but as the 'diazepam' began to kick in I entered the hazy world of modern medicine. A green barley cocktail with a milligram of paracetamol washed it all down and by ten o'clock I was floating across Malaga's Larios Square, heading to the Medibio Clinic for the next round.

The team were pleased with what seemed to be happening with the breast, having not seen me for over a month. They set to work hooking me up and I fell asleep for an hour and a half, since I had only managed an hour or two the night before. Waking up to the dreaded waves of electricity pulsing through my body brought tears of frustration, and I decided almost immediately that I would have them stop right there and then. I was ready to take my chances…enough was enough!

Doctora Maridoxia with her usual bright and positive countenance calmed me down and lowered the voltage so that I could manage another hour. The last thirty minutes seemed like an eternity and I again wanted to stop it, but she kept insisting that I had come this far; it didn't make sense to quit now.

~ And So We Heal ~

Another five milligrams of diazepam was slipped under my tongue and by the grace of God the next thing I remember is the bell going off to signal that the session was over. Laurent came in to unhook me and I asked what the reading was on the machine.

"300!"

A flashing light went off inside my mind-everything was in a slower than usual motion...

300 was the magic number. This is what I had been waiting to hear for the last six months. Some invisible force was finally indicating that I had reached a zenith with its protocol, and from far away a distant whisper chanting across the heavens - ***'It's gone, it's gone!'***

300 means cancer-free!

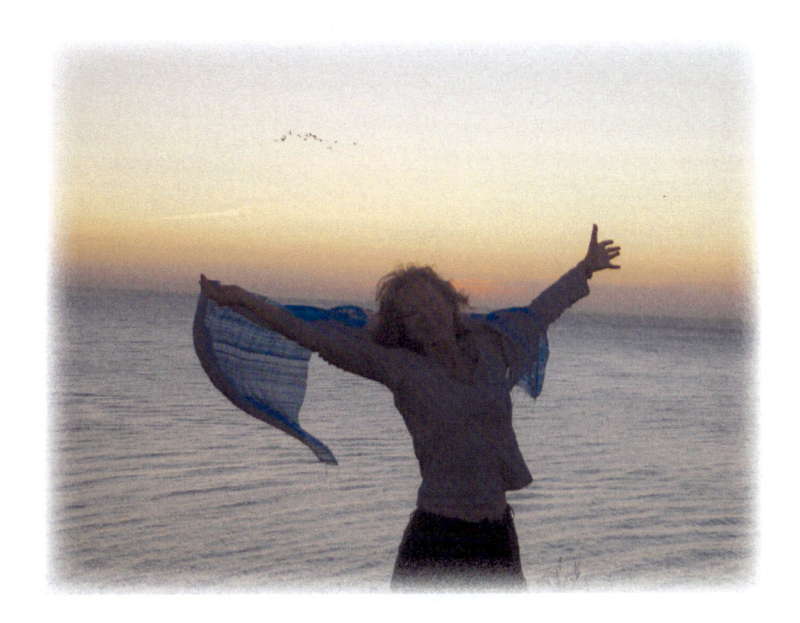

Chapter Twelve

It's Gone

> "An empowered spirit is capable of healing a diseased body."

Since I had not travelled the orthodox route with my treatments, there was no one telling me that I was in 'remission' as they say. Certainly the BET/ECT machine had signalled an 'all clear' physically at that moment in time, but it was wishful thinking that a bell could go off and that's it – 'healing complete'. I knew that cancer leaves its impression in the psyche – we needed to get the message through to all the cells that the war is over, so to speak.

To monitor my progress more accurately Laurent had wanted me to move to Malaga for an extended period so that I could take full advantage of the Papimi machine and also some special Crystal Water designed by Doctor Dolores Del Rio from Mexico that he had been having success with.

He was right in that I needed to continue with a follow-up regime, but as always, I had to follow my inner voice, and felt that spending time with Javier in Barcelona and also my mother who herself was not in good health, was just as important to my well being. Instead I would continue to travel back and forth as time and money allowed.

February 24, 2006, Andalucia
It's time to check the breast again.

~ And So We Heal ~

I arrived in Malaga yesterday on the usual early morning flight. It wasn't easy pulling myself away from Javier, It's been sweet staying with him, watching him paint and move forward with his life. His studio is a small space for two and can be quite challenging, but these days I acknowledge a shift in my well-being.

I believe that the tumour came as a messenger, and when it left, it took with it a lot of the heaviness; the excess baggage, I was carrying for so long.

Finally I am beginning to feel more the person I once was, but with a new strength to uphold my values.

At the Medibio Clinic, M. Eudoxia examined my breast noting that although there does seem to be a hard 'knobble' still there at the side, the tissue surrounding it is much softer and my blood tests indicate that the liver is in good shape. I have a session on the 'Papimi' machine, and take the late bus up in to the mountains to Los Ventorros to see Ruth. It's freezing cold, but Ruth welcomes me in to 'El Duende' with hot tea and a roaring fire around which we catch up on life. I know so many of her friends and neighbours by now and feel blessed by our friendship over the years. She truly is a pioneer spirit, with a story to fill volumes. By ten o'clock I am tucked up in bed and for the most part stay there until ten the next morning. A breakfast of fresh pineapple, soaked sunflower, and flax seeds, and figs; a nice hot bath, and I'm off up the mountain to Comares. It feels liberating to forgo the usual coffee enema that has been my daily ritual for years now. I am slowly trying to adapt my regime to present circumstances since it's virtually impossible to keep up, especially the juicing, when I travel so much.

I am trying so hard to become a 'normal' person, and forget that there was ever this thing called 'cancer'. The doctors still want me to do a PET scan, to assess the rest of my body. Of course I know it makes sense and I am awaiting the Okay from the NHS. They've already turned me down once, because I haven't followed their usual protocol, I suppose. I'm trying to argue the point that I would have cost the system a fortune by now. As it is I am still paying off the ECT treatment and am always in debt. But enough of that!

There is a bird singing joyfully in my heart, and it sings not of fear and sadness, but of all the dreams I once held precious. It calls to me now to have the courage to move forward with my life, make it all happen.

And so I continued trying hard to finish this book, but soon realised that working on it, especially using the computer, took its toll on my health so I was caught in a catch 22, since the book needed to be typed up. God bless my sister Barbara, who despite her own ill health at the time, offered to type up my diaries - without that there would have been no hope of continuing. Still, it was me that needed to pull the whole thing together, and trying to do so in the midst of what now seemed like the onset of menopause would trigger yet another healing acceleration. I kept thinking about Dr. Hamer's theory and the many stages of healing. How was one to know when the conflict was truly resolved?

Even though I felt that I had resolved the conflict, in many ways, there was still the issue of the psyche, and until all my cells got the message there was still work to do.

Painting my angels and inspirational touchstones, took the place of writing for a while. Wherever I went it seemed that people were in some kind of need.

I longed to be back to this 'normal', that everyone referred to, but as time went by I realised that I was never ever going to find normal again. So I'd best set my sights a little higher!

Chapter Thirteen
Cultivating the Power to Survive

> Suffering is the sister of your future possibility. Suffering can open a window in the closed wall of your life and allow you to glimpse the new pastures of creativity on which you are called to walk and wander…
> John O´Donahue

January 31, 2007, Barcelona

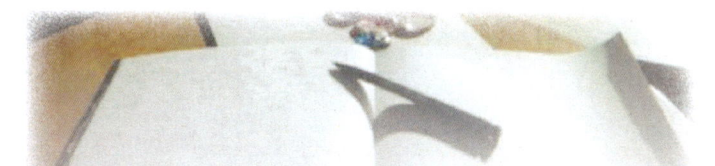

It's been months since I've written in my diary or anywhere for that matter. Words that once flowed easily now topple out with syllables missing and sentences rail against making the page. But hey, here I am again putting pen to paper. Let's see where the adventure takes me.

I am still going back and forth between England and Spain where I continue, as best I can, with my healing.

It's good to be back in Barcelona and snuggling up to Javier at night brings equilibrium to my being. I feel that I have come full circle these past seven years, and now I have promised myself to finish the book that I actually started when I arrived in 2000; albeit a much different love story from the one I had originally envisioned.

May 18, 2007, UK
Whilst in Barcelona I had a heavy period after three months without one, and my cancer markers are slightly elevated so I am assuming it's all to do with fluctuating hormone levels...

I had acupuncture at the Baozhlin Chinese Medicine Clinic in the village of Moreton. The treatment included stomach and head massage and a strong herbal mixture designed to aid menopause-Yep-Finally, 'la menopausia' – At least something's got me writing again!

May 28, 2007, UK
The blood seems to have lessened today...seven days in total. I am wondering if it had anything to do with the Chinese herbs, as I am sure they have 'Dong Quai' in them, which boosts oestrogen, and perhaps, given my circumstances, I am best off without it; although later down the line I'm sure it could benefit. Just my intuition, but lets face it, that's pretty much all I have these days.

In an attempt to halt any further growth to the lesions that are still persisting around the scars, I've been putting on a poultice of turmeric, green clay, and castor oil. As a result, the wound is red raw and suppurating with yellowness seeping out, so part of me thinks I need to continue, as turmeric is powerful and has great healing properties to shrink tumour, but on the other hand the pain factor from the burning will be an issue. Thank God for the local district nurse, Irene, or Luvvy duvvy as I endearingly call her. She keeps me going with plenty of swabs and dressings and a bright positive countenance every time I see her. Apparently often after mastectomy women get these re-occurrences popping up, and it's quite a common problem. Photo-dynamic therapy, PDT has proved successful in many cases, but since I have not heard anything from the NHS regarding my request for 'PDT, I need to move forward with other plans.

Laurent still wants me to return to Malaga to 'finish it' as he puts it. He is right; I did not follow through, as I needed to, because of my limited finances. There's been so much going on, and I hoped that the lesions would just fade away.

Come October 25th, it will be six years. If I had gone the traditional route I would probably be facing secondaries now, a term referring to the cancer returning, so I count myself lucky that although the breast looks pretty awful at the moment, everything is on the surface where I can see it. Thank God nothing has spread anywhere else, and God willing all this activity with my menstruation is simply part of the menopause.

I leave for Spain in ten days, and if nothing has come through about the 'PDT', I will go to Malaga and do another round of 'fire' with the ECT. It's not surprising that it is all circling the summer solstice yet again.

Talking of fire...I've been taking the homeopathic remedy Diospyros Kaki for the last month - 'Japanese Persimmon', survival tree as it is known, found after the nuclear fallout at Nagasaki. It symbolises light, detoxifies, and is associated with 'survival-revival'-
The power to survive.
DIO= ZEUS (GOD)
SPYROS = SPIRIT/SOUL
Dios, meaning God, Fruit of the Gods, Divine fruit.
KA = Soul
KI = Energy, earth. In Japan there used to be a deep religious connection to the Kaki, with life. Given as an offering on Shinto shrines. The kaki has a tradional relationship to life, death, the souls of the ancestors and the nameless dead, as is the case in wartime. It survived the deadly destruction of the plutonium bomb. Plutonium, the deadly destroyer
Diospyros Kaki- survival - revival of hope.

In the Edda (800-1000 BC north Germanic and Scandinavian mythology) Yggdrsil is the tree of the world. It connects Heaven and Earth.

Since Dr. Richardson has retired, my new homeopath Dr. Hayhurst thought that it may apply to my temperament, and indeed I think it may have some significance to my Japanese connection. So much of my purification has been through fire.

May 31, 2007, UK

The storytellers of all tribes and nations are the bridge to other times and ancient teachings. The children of future generations learn from the storytellers and apply lessons of the medicine stories to their own lives.

I re-remember my role as 'storyteller' and how my experience of healing my breast is important to tell.

No matter how difficult it is to get these words out – I will not give up! I must take a stand.

June 20, 2007, Barcelona

It's been two weeks ago now since I arrived back in Barcelona. Javier met me at the airport and we picked up where we left off, two peas in a pod, one always rolling off somewhere. That would seem to be me! Time went all too quickly and then the inevitable roll back to Andalucia. It's been such a part of my agenda these past years for my treatment and this time I really fought against it, but ultimately, felt I needed to take some form of action again.

I arrived yesterday afternoon and a taxi sped me off into yet another unknown. Laurent has let me use his guesthouse up in Los Pinares de San Anton. It's a wonderful location high in the mountains overlooking

~ And So We Heal ~

the sea. Wheels are really essential but a local bus conveniently picks up every half hour. Simone, his beautiful wife and son Sebastian, greet me with open arms, and after preparing a good meal I sleep like a baby.

In the morning I take the early bus into Malaga for my appointment with Doctora Eudoxia. She seems to think that the breast is in good shape but we both agree I should have another ECT on Friday. Hopefully one will do it. Meanwhile I can get PAPIMI every day and hopefully get back to writing. I've taken the afternoon bus to El Palo, and sit watching the waves. The beach is not the best and it's quite evident that the murky water is not suitable to bathe in, but the negative ions in the air are a lift to the spirit.

June 23, 2007, Andalucia

I'm Sitting on the beach at El Palo with the aftermath of last night's celebrations for el dia de St Juan, and the annual fires. I actually missed out on seeing the grand fires ablaze over Spain. Yesterday at nine thirty a.m. I had my ECT treatment and by the time I got back to my mountain retreat, sleep was the main order of the day.

Once again the ECT was not easy to bear. It's the initial needles going in that provoked the first tears, a mixture of fear and memory, ancient memory really, but nothing that hasn't already been laid to rest. More a case of fearful anticipation of what was to come. When the electricity began it was uncomfortable and three hours seemed a long, long way away. I was given some pain medication in a drip plus the usual diazepam, and with that I enter the familiar hazy zone.

Three hours do pass and I'm home free. Removing the needles and padding the wound with betadine, stings provoking a few more tears. I wander into the hot afternoon sun seeking reward. Sustenance comes in the form of a vegetable wok creation with the inevitable over-excitement of sodium but I waffle it down hungrily and follow it up with a lemon ice cream, a pitiful portion really that disappears quickly, then off to catch the bus to El Palo. The bus is late and I miss my connection up to the eagle's lair; but a taxi is only five Euro and there's even time to purchase a couple of bottles of Asturian cider, so I treat myself... Apples..........mmmmmmmmmm...This is the kind of natural pain medicine for me! Apparently they are doing scientific testing on the amazing benefits of natural cider.

After a two-hour siesta I head back into the village to make a few phone calls almost missing the last bus up again. The evening finds me painting, what else but an angel, which I am going to give to the Medibio Clinic as a way of saying thank you. By midnight I'm in bed envisioning all the folk along the coast partaking of the annual leaping – over-fire, and dipping- into-the-ocean ritual.

June 30, 2007

It's nine-thirty pm. and I'm on the sleeper train from Malaga to Barcelona, sipping on a nice glass of Rioja whilst rolling through the dusky sunset between these two cities. I've actually seen so very little of Spain over these last six years... it's all been travelling for healing. Since I made my mind up at the last minute to travel back by train, I am enjoying the fringe benefits of this 'movie' from the window; colours of the landscape changing constantly, lolling back and forth with my fellow diners. What's the point in travelling this way if one can't enjoy a bit of luxury. 'Ahhh'...so delightful to sit like this, pen in hand, observing the comings and goings of those around me, and the waiter, a handsome soul making me blush with his attentive nature. "Senora this", and "Senora that!" I've been very much of a recluse lately and apart from my one lunch with friends this is the first meal out since my arrival. I never even got to partake of my favourite skewered sardines, at the beach. What is the world coming to!

~ And So We Heal ~

Anyway, here I am rolling back to Barcelona. I've learned a lot about myself these last few days. I've fought off loneliness, and I've created art. The journey continues to regain my health, with the elements always conspiring to bring about these somewhat off the beaten track experiences. I am so grateful…

> By the love of God,
> I feel that I am saved,
> and that this salvation
> is for me to help others in some way.

It's past ten o'clock and the dusky sunset has faded into an evening blue. Someone has just come to tell me that my bed has been made and since the wine bottle is empty and I have no companion to share my gratitude with, it's time to lay the head down and dream. Methinks tomorrow is July!

July 5, 2007, Barcelona

I arrived back into the arms of Javier and we spent blissful times curled up after making love. It truly felt like we had crossed a bridge in our lives, at times the light flooding in and through us. During orgasm I could feel a sense of re-birth, somehow feeling very much part of the ocean. More and more I appreciate the role that the sexual energy has to play in healing. I am grateful for this and am reminded of the message in the Sacred Path Card, 'Thunder Beings'-

'We humans are catalysers who have electromagnetic, giving and receiving bodies. Like Mother Earth and Father Sky we are male and female in nature.'

Did I say 'thunder'?
  It's hard to believe, but in the space of the last twenty-four hours

~ And So We Heal ~

everything has fallen apart and we've reached ground zero yet again. It's all over some silly argument about how to cook rice. We've got our different methods you see, and suddenly it was 'boom! We both exploded. I as always wanted to drop it straight away and carry on as if it was all silly nonsense, but Javier reacts differently and has retreated into his darkness, refusing to accept middle ground. I spent the night in a wounded state, hoping that the bright light of day would find him changed. It was not to be. I spent the next day alone and went for a Ceragem session of infra red light and massage that I had found. Can you imagine a daily forty minute session completely gratis.

As I relaxed I found myself opening up to one of the assistants there who was talking to me. Funny how complete strangers can push the necessary buttons to release the pain. My breast had been feeling quite inflamed yesterday as I think I overdid it with the infrared, so all in all feeling sad and irritable; the usual signs leading up to the parting from Javier again, knowing that I would miss him…many things really all connected to the healing.

It's all about release and once I let the tears out I felt better *and took myself walking through the streets trying to not think of this rupture with Javier, knowing that if I just leave him be, all will eventually pass over. It will just take time.*

In times when I've needed to pull back from certain situations and take a deep breath, It's been so helpful to have the help of these Oracles such as *The Sacred Path Cards* and the *'Runes'*. They inevitably offer peace of mind. Picking the Runes to see what is going on I draw:

~ And So We Heal ~

WUNJO - JOY AND LIGHT- it is a fruit-bearing branch and signifies the term of travail has ended.

You have come into yourself in some regard.
The shift that was due has occurred,
and now you can freely receive the blessings.

Light pierces the clouds and touches the waters just as something lovely emerges from the depths. The soul is illuminated from within at the meeting place of heaven and Earth, the meeting of the waters. It is the rune of, self properly aligned to self.

Self aligned to self…know thyself.

The message I gleaned was that Javier and I needed to let each other 'be'. It was as simple as that. I was finally learning how to get on with my life, and leaving him to get on with his own 'stuff'. It was painful sometimes, but it was no longer life-threatening. And guess what? In this way we usually met in the middle somewhere, and everyone was happy.

July 21, 2007, UK

Last night's dream, equally as simple…
Javier and I were beneath the sheets, giggling happily amidst a cloud of smoke.

The Sacred Path card SMOKE SIGNALS comes to mind, teaching us that the Red Race has understood and utilised many unspoken languages for centuries. Reading the signs in the faces in the clouds, changes in weather, messages in our medicine dreams, language of the heart, etc, Communication - Bridge between Heaven and Earth - smoke forms are one way in which spirit can be visually seen by human kind -True Freedom is to be found by those that find illumination through the truth that lives inside their hearts.

and more...

A few nights ago my dream was simple yet clear.
A tray of plain white A4 pages of paper slid into my consciousness.
I can only interpret it as one thing -The Book.
It's now or never...
I shall complete this.

September 11, 2007... 9/11
(Twenty minutes to touchdown in Malaga)
I've just spent the last week with Javier. As always, time goes all too quickly and goodbye yet again. We had a nice peaceful time together and shared some deeper thoughts on life. Not that either of us really knows what lies ahead, but at least we still come together and touch each other in special places.

I got good results with the blood tests and my cancer markers are back to normal.

The 'PET Scan' however (having finally arranged one) was inconclusive as it was taken too close to the time I did ECT.

The really good news is that the swollen lymph node under the arm that I have had for over five years did not show up on the scan, and indeed seems to have disappeared. Ms. Waghorn is quite amazed. Laurent is suggesting that we do more ECT, finish the job as he's fond of saying, but I really had hoped to avoid it, and still hope that Dr. Eudoxia will say that the breast is doing fine and I can just do 'Papimi' instead. We'll see.

Meanwhile my dream a few nights ago brought two cranes flying high in the sky, signifying happiness, and below them two magpies...Joy!

Now if that's not the perfect omen, I don't know what is.

December 10, 2007, El Duende, Andalucia

Before I left Barcelona I had a dream of a beautiful white tree. When I stood underneath it and looked up into its branches they had transformed into white horses... magnificent actually...Horses symbolising success.

I arrived in Malaga last Tuesday evening, and decided not to do any more ECT treatment. My body is now instinctively saying a definite 'no'.

The 'Papimi' however feels really good and empowering, so this trip combines a few things. The mountains have called me and it feels good to get away from the noise of Barcelona. I came to spend a week with Ruth at El Duende. The weather here is perfectly warm and the energy as always feels good. I spend time mulling over the contents of the book and fulfil a dream to ride a horse again, with a full fearless gallop - how could I not after such a powerful dream.

Taking this time to return to El Duende is a completion of sorts, bringing my healing to a closure. I'm feeling more centred about my 'core being', and getting used to having just the one breast, although I still envision growing another somehow. For now, I'm just happy to be alive and in good health; continuing with a healthy regime that includes drinking green barley juice every day and a substantial amount of vitamins, including 'adaptogenos', recommended by Laurent at Medibio. I'm still injecting Iscador, mistletoe, and occasionally taking various other homeopathic remedies, which I will no doubt continue with as a boost to my immune system.

~ And So We Heal ~

The smells and the sounds of nature intoxicate my world, as warm sunshine infuses the day. I am embraced by an endless symphony of chickens clucking, wild birds singing, goat bells tinkling, and, bees buzzing, and from far across the valley echoes of a solitary broom sweeping away the dust of yesterday… Six years have come and gone and now as I enter into the seventh year I am determined to do so leaving the past behind me.

The cells in my body feel as if they are renewing themselves following a kind of decoding, a de-programming, if you will, from any negative connections to the past...

Everything feels like it's 'yet to be' - alive with an inspired hope. I'm painting again, angels as always, and lots of butterflies this time, grateful for the magic and ever sensitive to the 'duende' gently whispering to my soul.

It takes me back to one of the many dreams during my separation from Javier in America 2001, when I was searching for an answer to understand the darkness that I had fallen into.

In the dream, two brightly coloured butterflies appeared to come together and kiss each other whereupon a bright star burst between them, waking me up, with the definite message that Javier and I would indeed be re-united - one day.

It came as an omen, which would only show its true significance years later in 2006. I was in Mexico to see Dr Dolores del Rio at her clinic, Therese Dilor in search of 'Crystal water' (see appendix) While I was there, Javier suggested I visit the great pyramids of 'Teotijuacan', even though they were hours away and I had to take a taxi. It was another unbelievable journey that found me climbing the pyramid of the sun. As I reached the summit, somewhat breathless, I lifted my head to find two giant monarch butterflies dancing together, immediately connecting me back to that dream.

~ And So We Heal ~

I love this passage from Deepak Chopra's writing; having so often been uplifted by his wisdom:

(Birth of a butterfly)
Biologists tell us that in the tissue of a caterpillar there are embedded cells that they call imaginal cells. They resonate at a different frequency. They are so unlike the other caterpillar cells that the worm's immune system thinks they are the enemy and tries to destroy them. But the new imaginal cells continue to appear, more and more of them. Eventually the caterpillars' immune system cannot destroy them fast enough and they become stronger, they connect, and connect until they form a critical mass that realises their mission to bring about the amazing birth of a butterfly.

As I began to contemplate this miracle of transformation and how I might apply it to my own rebirth, I began to envision the healthy cells inside my body as the imaginal cells, fighting to transform the old me, whilst the cancer cells fighting to take over, gradually were defeated. I cannot repeat enough this thing about the mind being the final frontier, and how very important it is to…

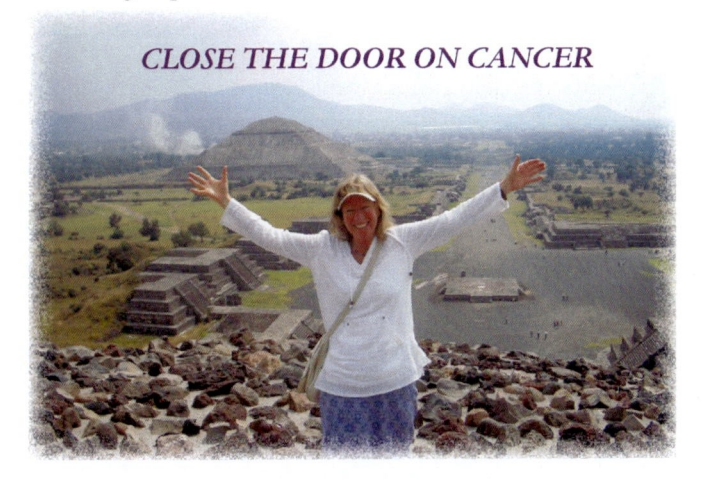

CLOSE THE DOOR ON CANCER

~ And So We Heal ~

Chapter Fourteen

Closing the Door on Cancer

> Where there is a wound on the bodies and psyches of women, there is a corresponding wound at the same site in the culture itself, and finally on Nature itself.
>
> 'Women who run with Wolves'
> Clarissa Pinkola Estés

Determined to keep the door closed I begin 2008 with a stronger than ever determination to find a 'new beginning'. Reading *Women Who Run With Wolves* by Clarissa Pinkola Estés was pure gold. Even though I had for many years, known of this amazing book I am sorry to say that I did not begin to fully devour its contents until this stage in my life, but finding it again was like finding the hidden treasure at the end of a long, long search. In it, she writes of the significance, especially to women's lives of stories, and fairytales, handed down over the ages. In the old traditions it is the balm of these 'miracle stories', 'cuentas de milagros', that is applied. In prayerful 'curandisima', they are considered encouragement, advice, and resolution.

With references to 'canto hondo', the deep song, and 'hambre del alma', the starved soul, she explains that over time through experience, dreams and women's own wild life force, a force rises to the surface of the psyche, and breaks out the necessary cry, the cry that frees.

Finding fragments of myself and others within so many of these stories, and recognizing my own story as something that may help others in their search to heal I was finally able to honour the last seven years as a true gift.

It was finally time to close the door on this chapter of my life.

Needing safe and fertile ground to give it birth, where better to turn then than to an old American artist friend, Michele Thyne whom I first met in Hollywood. She was now living in Italy.

22/2/2008, Umbria, Italy
Breathing in this Italian paradise, I am reminded of how inspired I was one afternoon, in Barcelona in 2001, months before my diagnosis, reading Frances Mayes book, 'Under the Tuscan Sun' fantasizing then of creating my new life in Europe. As fate would have it, whilst my journey took me off in another direction, Michele it would seem beat me to the gate, and renovated an old barn in the Umbrian countryside. What a joy now to behold the absolute splendour that she has created, much with her own hands, within these magical walls. To be welcomed as a sister and to finally have this time to give priority to the book in such a glorious abode is truly a miracle.

Sitting outside in a fresh invigorating breeze I can hear the sound of bells softly tinkling throughout her beautiful garden. Rufus, her majestic wolf-like companion, and Sofia the devoted new puppy, stand guard at my feet. Birds sing and there's a mysterious croaking in the air. Is it frogs I wonder, or some winged creatures, come to herald the whispers of el duende once again?

Embraced by this incessant wonder of nature I am finally able to reach out and grasp the golden thread… I must draw it in now; weave

~ And So We Heal ~

an ending to this tapestry of words.

Amongst Michele's collection of books I find a copy of my own "Bridges a Memoir of Love." Ironically in perusing through some of the pages I am drawn back towards Hollywood again and my experience on the film 'The Bridges of Madison County'. A simple glance at my reflection in the mirror, and I suddenly find Francesca the Italian housewife, the character that Meryl played so beautifully. Francesca's character is perhaps a symbol for all the broken dreams I left behind in Hollywood.

Memory finds me seated at the table to re-enact the last scene with Clint. He had wanted to re-do his close-up and since Meryl had already finished filming and returned home, he asked me to be the voice of Francesca and feed him the lines... Of course nobody would be seeing any of this on the big screen, but I had no choice as a professional other than to give it my all anyway.

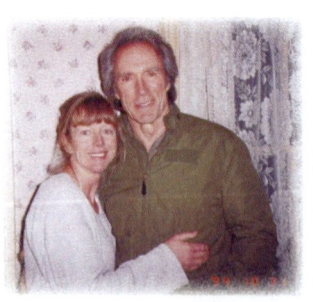

I was the guinea pig to test Meryl's "old age" make-up today.

The fun part was making myself cry so they could determine how well the process would hold up under stress. Meryl has a lot of emoting to do

The tears kept coming for at least another half hour, but they became my own as I began to dig up all sorts of sad memories buried in the archives of my heart. I guess in a way I was taking the

"We are the choices we have made," I tell him, Italian accent somehow falling effortlessly from my mouth....

Choices...There it was... ...whispering to me again...twelve years later.

Quite unbelievable to think of the twists and turns my life has taken. And yes indeed...this journey for me has been all about the choices I made...even those I made before I was diagnosed with cancer. The choice I made to stop pursuing my career as an actress for example; after so many years of dedication.

~ *And So We Heal* ~

Was I really O.K. with all that now...or was there still some part of me that thought I had given up, when really I should have carried on believing in my dream?

I find the answer within the tattered file of 'this and that' I hurriedly packed...research material, photos, poems, etc. It was written on an old notepad, previously stored away in my mother's attic gathering dust with all my old Hollywood memorabilia...

June 15, 1992, Los Angeles, California

I am back on the set of 'Death Becomes Her', standing in for Meryl.

Dear God,

Thank you for bringing Javier back into my life when I needed him the most. I can hardly believe my feelings for him. I love him so much and yet we have these separate lives. If I could make a wish right now it would be to wake every morning in his arms. I don't know what the future will bring, I only know that I cannot run away, because then I will have given up.

When I think back to Ibiza and watching him from my window and knowing then that I wanted him twenty-one years ago, and now all this time has passed between us — all the experiences, the memories.

Somehow I am willing to let go of everything for him.

What kind of person am I to be able to live this life?

Will I ever really know myself?

I have a dream to make films about the human spirit - I must take this next step with my life - I must bridge this gap somehow.

Dear God give me the strength to endure. Keep Javier safe, and if there be a way, bring him back in my arms forever. He is the man I love and will always love...

There I was still talking to God even then...

It all came back to me... how determined I was to be successful with my acting, how very hard I tried... I was courageous enough to follow my dreams and made my way to Hollywood in pursuit of them. I was successful to a certain degree I suppose, although I never found the kind of fame or fortune that I once equated with success. However in reflection, I now understand that instead of making a living as an actress playing characters that fight for noble causes, with this diagnosis, I've actually become one of those characters who are championing change. Instead of merely acting out those roles, I have actually been living a very full life, rich with beauty, experience and inspiration. But what touches me most of all is how much I loved. In that, I never gave up, and that's what really counts.

I never did give up believing after all…

As I said at the beginning…there are many paths to healing. I simply wanted to feel good about my choices. That is why I wrote this book really…in the hope that my story could inspire others with their choices.

As my story has told, Javier and I were slowly drawn back together, but not before being plunged into the fire. Over these past eight years since reuniting we have worked hard to overcome many obstacles; and since he is a much more private person than I, it is my story told within these pages, my take on this long odyssey to finally accept and know myself. Javier has his own story, much of it expressed through the paintbrush and not the pen, although he himself writes passionately every day.

~ *And So We Heal* ~

Through the years, ever the romantic, part of me has held on to the concept of everlasting love, and I am proud of that choice as ultimately it did indeed play a major part in weaving me back together...

I am reminded of how one afternoon last week as Javier and I lay together, I began tracing the scar over his heart, with my finger, and suddenly realised that part of the scar on my chest appears to have a similar configuration, and then without thinking too much about it I slipped off my top and for the first time in a long while, perhaps two years - I exposed my wound. It was something I had wanted to do many times before but Javier was not ready, as he still has painful memories of his own heart surgery, but in that moment he was. It felt very liberating after all this time, and later making love, there were sweet tears of dissolution at play.

I have no doubt that Javier and I came together to heal deep wounds, and in this we have succeeded. There was indeed an ocean of tears that needed to be shed...

There are oceans of tears women have never cried, for they have been trained to carry mother's and father's secrets, men's secrets, society's secrets, and their own secrets, to the grave. A woman's crying has been considered quite dangerous; for it loosens the locks and bolts on the secrets she bears. But in truth, for the sake of a woman's wild soul, it is better to cry. For women, tears are the beginning of initiation into the Scar Clan, that timeless tribe of women of all colours, all

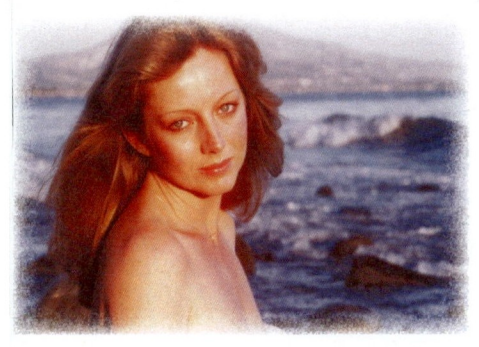

~ And So We Heal ~

nations, all languages, who down through the ages have lived through a great something, and yet who stood proud, still stand proud...The fact is that for women and men, woundings to the self, soul, and psyche through secrets and otherwise, are part of most persons' lives.
Neither can the subsequent scarring be avoided. But there is help for these injuries, and absolutely there is healing.'

Women Who Run With Wolves

ABSOLUTELY THERE IS HEALING...

Yet another title to consider and the book may have ended here, but since I had spent so much of this journey delving through open portals, I find it difficult now to close the door on this final chapter when there still seems so much more to say...

Within the pages of this book I have tried to be as honest and open as possible with my feelings.

Holistic healing is something that can no longer be denied – many many people are finding ways to heal outside of the current 'system'.

Just as our political and financial systems are coming under scrutiny for their abuse against the common decent man, surely it is time to take our own lives in hand and demand that we the people are given more humane choices to find wellness, without being forced to endure a lifetime of toxic medicine to further fill the coffers of the pharmaceutical fat cats.

There are many well-documented books on healing cancer holistically, some of which I list in the appendix, so I've tried to focus instead on the importance of the emotional healing

~ And So We Heal ~

– the healing of the human heart, and thereby encourage others to speak out, and live their lives courageously and creatively.

…And so…with both an ending and new beginning in sight I endeavour to put together a cover…The images that manifest remind me of yet another dream, a beautiful dream I had one night a few years ago when all seemed lost:

I was standing in the ocean naked attended by some women who were attempting to drape a greenish gold shawl over me, when Javier appeared and took over the task, placing the shawl, which was soaked by the water around me.

Coincidently knowing nothing about this dream, Javier's mother, Sofia presented me with a beautiful green and gold shawl this year and once again I am reminded of the message of 'the taking of the shawl' - how it marks the road back to finding the heart of spirit - to acknowledging the beauty in each unique expression of creation.

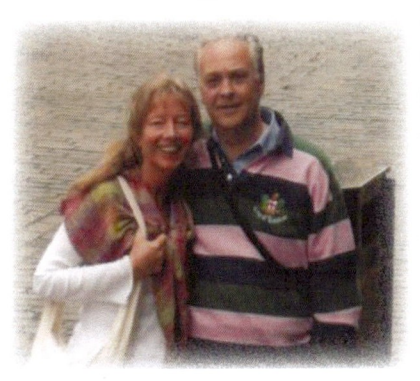

Coming home to the magic that we once believed in…

Love

…And so we heal…

~ And So We Heal ~

Epilogue

October 2009

As fate would have it, Bush has finally left the White House, all my blood tests are showing normal, Meryl has wowed us in "Mamma Mia", and por Dios I have finally finished this book!

~ And So We Heal ~

BIBLIOGRAPHY

Quantum Healing, Deepak Chopra, Bantam, Dell, Pub. Group
Women Who Run with Wolves, Clarissa Pinkola Estés, Ballantine
Anatomy Of The Spirit, Carolyn Myss, Harmony Books
Anam Cara, Eternal Echoes, John O'Donahue, Bantam Books
An Offering of Light, Roy Gibbon & Atsushi Fujimaki, Shumei America Publications
Heal Your Life, Louise L.Hays, Hay House
Sacred Path Medicine Cards, Jamie Sams, Harper Collins
Back to Eden, Jethro Kloss
A Cancer Therapy, Max Gerson MD, The Gerson Institute, San Diego, CA
Healing, The Gerson Way, Charlotte Gerson, Beata Bishop
German New Medicine, Dr. Ryke Geerd Hamer, www.newmedicine.com
Salves That Heal, Ingrid Naiman
Cancer As Initiation, Barbara Stone
The Alchemist, Paul Coelho, Harper Collins
The Emerald Tablet, Dennis William Hauck, Penguin
Last night I dreamed, (poem) Antonio Machada
The Bridges of Madison County, James Robert Waller, Warner Books

APPENDIX – UK & Europe:

Jyorei – for centre listings - www.shumei.org
Wirral Holistic Cancer Services, 6 Ashburton Rd, Claughton,(01516529313) www.wirralholistic.org
Liverpool Dept. of Homeopathic Medicine, Old Swan Health Close, Liverpool, (01512853707)
The Linda Mc Cartney Clinic, Royal Liverpool Hospital,
Alan Hudson, Herbalist, 28 Moreton Rd, Upton, Wirral
Baozhlin Chinese Medicine, Emilian Chen, Moreton, Wirral: (151 678 8373)
The Penny Brohn Cancer Care Centre, www pennybrohncancercare.com
The Breast Cancer Haven, www.breastcancerhaven.org.uk
The Dove Clinic, Hampshire, (01962712226) www.doveclinic.com
Debra Stappard Trust, Chapel Farm, West Humble,Dorking ,Surrey, RH 56AY,(01372817652)

~ And So We Heal ~

Rudolph Steiner, www.steinerinstitute.org
Macmillan Cancer Help, www.macmillan.org.uk
The Clouds Trust, Hampshire, (01730301162) www.cloudstrust.org
Lukas Clinic, Switzerland, www.lukasklinic.com, (41-0617020909)
Rainforest, Fair-trade ethnic, new age music &books, 51 Watergate Row, Chester, (01244340200)
www.papimi.com/ *Professor* Pannos Pappos

SPAIN
Medibio Clinic,Malaga, Spain info@clinicamedibio.com -info@papimi.eu
Laurent Schidler "El cáncer no es ninguna enfermedad, sino un síntoma de incapacidad de regeneración ordenada de tus células, por desequilibrio de tu medio ambiente celular. No hay nada que combatir o destruir, salvo el síntoma si causa alguna molestia, y si se hace, nunca se debe de usar terapias agresivas, pues necesito cada órgano, cada célula de mi cuerpo....
Los tratamientos agresivos tales como los citotoxicos o radiaciones desequilibran áun mas el entorno celular, por lo tanto, son la causa de mas tumores. Si no se agrede el organismo y en vez de esto, se restablecen los elementos de base en un ser vivo, el síntoma conocido como tumor desaparecerá de la misma forma que ha aparecido... Para los lectores interesados, la base científica y las pruebas se ha publicado en FUNIBER, fundación iberomaricana (www.funiber.org), dentro de un Master en Medicina, y presentada en el I Congreso Internacional de Medicina y terapias alternatives." http://www.medicinasalternativas.com.ec/
El Duende, (Retreat) Los Ventorros, Comares, Andalucia, www.elduende.com
José Antonio Cruz Teruel, Spiritual healer, C/ Amigó, 49.1a (34696755502)
Libreria los Angeles, Travassera de Gracia, 157, Barcelona
Arunachala Libreria, C/Jovellanos 1, Barcelona

Recommended reading and research sources:

Your Life In Your Hands, Professor Jane Plant, Macmillan
Living Proof, Michael Gearin -Tosh, Simon & Schuster
A Time To Heal, Beata Bishop, Penguin
Everything You Need To Know About Cancer, Chris Woollams
Choosing to Heal, Janet Edwards, Watkins Publishing
The Journey, Brandon Bays, Harper Collins
The Cancer Prevention Book, Rosy Daniel, Rachel Ellis, Hunter House

~ And So We Heal ~

Gifts of the Spirit, Reflections, Ardath Rodale, www.prevention.com
Keep Your Breasts, Susan Moss, Re-Source Publications
A Slice of Life, Lee Sturgeon Day
Dr. Lorraine Day – www.drday.com
Sincerity and Truth, The Life Story of Meishusama, Gerard Rohlfing, Shumei America Publications
ICON Magazine, www.iconmag.co.uk / www.canceractive.com
Cygnus Review, www.cygnus-books.co.uk

USA & MEXICO
Jyorei: See www.shumei.org for centre listings
The Cancer Control Society- www.cancercontrolsociety.com
The Gerson Institute, San Diego, California
Optimum Health Institute, San Diego, California, (1-800993-4325) www.optimumhealth.org

Crystal water, http://www.theresedilor.com/esther.html Dr.Esther Del Rio.

Art Contribution

Cover : Pauline Lomas, includes -Sandro Boticelli 'Birth of Venus', and 'Seascape' by Javier Infanzón,
Deborah Lomas- pages-36, 67, 91, 182
Javier Infanzón – pages-15, 23. 41
Marta Cabeza – p119
Rosella Longinotti, p93 www.rosella-creations.co.uk,
Mary Englebricht p31
All other art by Pauline Lomas

For further information and to order this book –contact- palomas33@hotmail.com

About the Author

Born in the United Kingdom, Pauline Lomas is an artist, writer and actress. Her first book *Bridges, A Memoir of Love, (Veracity Press)* chronicled her experience working with Clint Eastwood, and Meryl Streep on the film, *The Bridges of Madison County.* During her years in Hollywood she was Barbra Streisand's stand-in on *The Prince of Tides,* and other film credits include *Testament, Bugsy,* and *All of Me.* She was the voice of Alicia Masters on the CBS animated series *The Fantastic Four*, and she wrote and produced the promotional video *Light and Love,* and *Hello to all the Children of the World.* Other writings include *The Gemstones*, an animated children's story. As an artist she has created a line of inspirational glass art which includes *'Chalices of Light' and 'Touchstones.'*